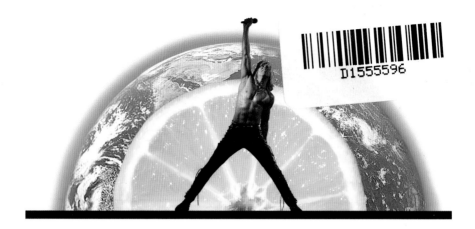

CONGRATULATIONS! YOUR LIFE IS ABOUT TO CHANGE

HEAL YOURSELF 101

Edition 3
by Markus Rothkranz

This information is a collection of studies, observations, research and practical advice written for the purposes of helping people help themselves become disease-free.

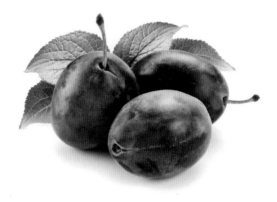

www.HealAnything.com

CONTENTS

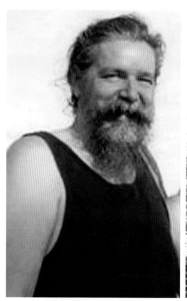 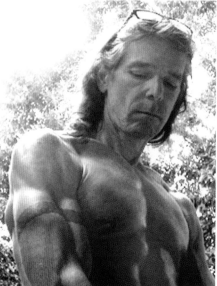

Before
48 year old
overweight vegetarian
Joseph Hill
/w.facebook.com/joseph.hill.veg

After
1 year later
following the raw food
lifestyle in this book

See more amazing testimonials at **MarkusMiracles.com**

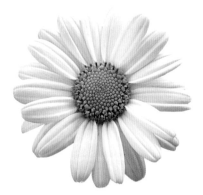

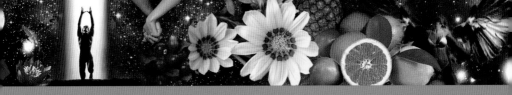

We were not born to die. We were born to live.

LIVING WAY PAST 100
BECOMING YOUNGER, SEXIER AND DISEASE FREE

THE HEALING STARTS NOW

What you will read in this book you will know is the truth.

PEOPLE EVERYWHERE ARE HEALING

If you have a serious disease or want to lose weight or get younger again, there is nothing on the planet that will get you there faster than what I am about to say in this book. It is simple. It costs very little, and you'll start seeing effects right away. The less you cheat, the more dramatic the effects will be.

My father had aggressive prostate cancer, his PSA was off the charts. He lived a life of meat, potatoes, bread and alcohol. We said to him: "Do you want to live? Are you willing to make a radical life change?" He said "yes" and within one month his cancer was completely GONE.

I've seen this lifestyle help people look 20 years younger and never get sick ever again. I know because I am one of them.

I have friends that got rid of things like polio and brain cancer (Jessie Bogdanovich, Bonnie Lovett). I've seen 400 lb diabetics get off insulin within DAYS. I've seen people lose 200 pounds (yes TWO HUNDRED POUNDS!!!) Google Philip McCluskey or Angela Stokes. I've seen what most would call miracles happen so regularly, I know without a doubt this works. It is simply going back to living the way nature designed us to live. That's all.

How do I know for sure what I'm saying is true? Because I've tried it on myself. I've interviewed people who healed themselves of life-threatening diseases. You should see some of the before-after pictures! Check out MarkusMiracles.com for a taste of what is possible when following this program. I don't care what any book or doctor says. I want to see and experience the results myself. Results speak for themselves.

Don't believe me. You need to try it yourself and watch what happens :-)

We are judged on the quality of our results, not on the quality of our excuses."

Steve Fargan

Truth always wins in the end. Let's not suffer or lose any more lives to realize this.

You will have to change some things in your life. You can't get better by continuing to do the things that made you sick.

Do what this book says, don't cheat, and I guarantee you will feel a difference. You will know that magic is really possible.

This is a life change and that scares some people. There is absolutely nothing to fear. Your life and food will NOT be more boring. In fact, you will feel a thousand times better. It definitely works but it requires will and staying power. Cooked and processed foods are addictive. Fear of change is the biggest factor.

As with any addiction, people start craving sugar, bread, pasta, cereal, pizza and cheese shortly after starting this cleanse and give up. The ones who hold tight then start to detox, and this process scares half of those people away because their bodies are bringing all kinds of crap to the surface that's been stored in their cells for years/decades. So now we are down to one quarter of the people that started. Their diseases go away. They feel great - SO great in fact, that they start to feel invincible and want to celebrate, so they go back to their old ways... they get sick, then go back to raw food again, feel better, celebrate by eating pizza, get sick, go back to healthy... and slowly over the years they start eating less bad and more good. This is a normal back and forth process where people try to see what they can get away with. Go ahead. It's a learning process.

"The intuitive mind is a sacred gift and the rational mind a faithful servant. We have created a society that honors the servant and has forgotten the gift."

Albert Einstein

This lifestyle definitely works... my allergies and asthma went away, my eyesight got better and I don't get sick anymore. It healed my dad's cancer. My business manager lost 40 lbs in the first 8 weeks. My friend Dean lost 210 lbs! Start with the basics and work your way from there. The main thing to start with is an awareness of what's right and wrong and then pay close attention to your body and how it reacts to what you do.

As you read this book, you will know it is the truth because it will resonate with you as something you always knew deep inside, but kept hidden in the corners. This truth has been nagging you quietly over the years and you knew one day you'd have to listen. That time is now. There is nothing to be afraid of. You will NOT lose comfort or lifestyle - as a matter of fact you will become an amazingly alive person who wishes they did this years or decades ago.

The sooner you start, the sooner you will be celebrating life like never before. What you will see in the mirror will be sexy and you'll forget what it was like to ever be sick.

THE TRUTH

The truth will set you free. It is insanely ridiculous that I have to write a book about this. This is like having to remind people that breathing is healthy.

What I am about to tell you is the most basic common sense that's been around since the beginning of time, and it boggles the mind how millions of people - especially in the modernized world, have forgotten this common sense to the point it seems foreign to them and something to fear and avoid.

What's even sillier, is this is nothing new. It's been like this for centuries. Sages heal people by reminding them of basic timeless natural laws. This isn't a profound magical secret, although to most caught up in the material rat race it seems that way. It's amazing that the little critters living just outside your house know more about health and longevity than you do, and they barely have a brain. Natural intuition is more powerful than all the rocket science in the world. As a species, we are the unhealthiest life form on the planet. We have been here the shortest amount of time and done the most damage. Actually we are the ONLY species causing damage. We are stressed-out materialistic comfort-driven beings totally out of touch with nature, and as a result hundreds of millions of people are rapidly aging, falling apart and dying long before their time. Almost everyone in the modern world has some kind of physical problem now. Many have silly diseases for no other reason than they are either too lazy or they just don't know any better. The motto is "I can do what I want, and if something happens, a doctor can fix it". Right? Wrong. Doctor's don't fix. They hide symptoms. They drug you up so you don't feel anything. They cut out infected body parts and give you poisons to try and kill things. If you break a bone or cut off a finger they put the bones and finger back in place and hope your body will heal it. Doctors don't heal you - your BODY does the healing. Ask a doctor what caused a disease and they probably won't have a clue.

If you had a disease, wouldn't you want to know what caused it, so you could stop doing it and make sure it didn't happen again?

The irony of the whole thing is we are "too busy" being in a hurry to be healthy or happy. We are so worried and concerned about racing the clock to get things done, that we are actually cutting our lives in half. We're trying to be efficient and save time, but in reality we are doing the opposite. If someone told you that you would live twice as long, wouldn't you start to take things a little easier? Wouldn't you take a little time to become healthier? Well that's exactly the case. The body you have been given is designed to live to at least 125. The Bible and many other religions even say that. A man in India just died who was 146. I met Bernando LaPallo who is 110 and outlived his son by 30 years... and he's still going strong! So my first message to you is: there is no need to hurry through your day. You have a long life ahead of you if you live the way you're designed. People, you live longer by slowing down! The longest living animals are turtles and elephants. STOP. Walk outside right now and look and take a deep breath. Feel the wind on your face. Look at the sky and listen to the birds. Now take your lover's hand and look in their eyes... REALLY look in their eyes. What do you see?

It's real simple. We are designed to function a certain way, and if we don't live that way, then trouble eventually arises. Everybody always says "what difference is one little soft drink or pizza or pasta going to make"? Firstly, it does not all come out of you the next day. Every molecule you put into your body is going to have an effect. Your body makes millions of new cells every minute and they use what's available at the time. That "one little" piece of unnatural comfort food becomes part of you. Those cells won't be able to properly absorb nutrients and expel waste like they are supposed to. Then the next day you'll have something else that's not totally raw and natural, again you say "this one little thing isn't going to make a difference in the long run". Again, 50 million more cells are made from inferior building materials, while others might even be harmed by the toxic nature of the snack. Most will be covered in mucus so they can't breathe... slowly suffocating. And on and on. You might not feel anything at first (just like termites that are secretly eating away your house), but pretty soon, these toxic little drops fill the bucket (your body) and you have a disaster.

"Nature is not negotiable, it's essential."

Dr. Ruza Bogdanovich

We are speeding down the highway of life. If we turn the steering wheel even one tiny half of a degree off center, we might stay on the road for a while, but eventually the car will run off the road and reality will hit us hard and fast. That is what our little "cheating" does. Don't think it's not leaving a mark. Look at how something that somebody told us many years ago can still stay with us in the back of our mind and still charge us emotionally today, even if that person is long gone. No difference. It's all energy. The energy effect of that donut or pizza or beer we had twenty years ago still reverberates in our cells. Everything leaves its mark. We can clean ourselves out mentally, physically and emotionally, but we will never again be the innocent, pure wide-eyed child we once were, who saw everything with fresh wonder and innocence. Sure we can learn to appreciate, but we will always be imbued with the underpinnings of life experience. The same goes for our body. We can clean it, heal it and make it healthy again, but it will have the energy scars of the past. That's why it's so important to do the right thing starting RIGHT NOW!

Whenever you find yourself on the side of the majority, it's time to pause and reflect."

Mark Twain

So enough of the doom and gloom. Yes, millions of people in the modern world are dying when not even halfway through their life. Almost all people in the modern world have some kind of health problem. Almost all of it can be avoided, reversed and healed. There are no guarantees, but if you are still alive, you have a serious fighting chance. I see what people call "miracles" every day. I got an email from a lady who survived pancreatic cancer because of this information. The only person who can heal you is YOU. The only way of doing it is following, honoring and obeying the natural laws of nature. If you honor mother nature, she will return the blessing and give you life - because that's what you were designed for.

This works. The only people who don't have some kind of results are those who are cheating or not following directions completely. It's human nature to see how much we can get away with. We all do it. Just be aware: you can't hide anything from nature or yourself.

Nature is non-judgmental. It doesn't care if you are rich or poor, young or old. If you follow natural law, you will be imbued with life. But those of you who cheat, be forewarned: for every action there is an opposite reaction. It is universal law. You can't cheat or beat nature. It always wins. You cannot eat bread, cheese, spaghetti, pizza, candy, drink alcohol and soft drinks, inhale cigarette smoke and expect to not pay for it. That's like those people who think they can cheat death by jumping off a crashing airplane at the last second just before it hits. No my friends, there are certain rules you must follow if you want to play this game right. Sure you can live it up and spend the last half of your life riddled with disease and discomfort, while the healthy people dance and play and laugh. Is that what you want? I am not going to kid you, because this is serious. Life or death. The choice is yours.

I want you to live. I want you to never get sick ever again. I want what you see in the mirror to get younger every day. I want you to know what it's like to be in a body that's so clean, you can feel things you never knew were possible. I want you to know what it's like to be orgasmic with every breath, every thought, every sound, smell and sight. You will never look at life the same way again, and feel a sense of peace you've never felt before. Imagine never feeling pain again. Imagine feeling naturally high and in tune with everyone everywhere. Imagine needing only a few hours of sleep and jumping out of bed at the first rays of the new day with the energy of a rocket. Imagine being filled with appreciation and love so vast you can feel the whole universe breathing and moving with you. Every step you take is like on coiled springs. Your heart is fully free and your body feels like that of a six-year-old. Your intuition is razor sharp and instantaneous because your brain is a supercomputer and your soul is channeling the voice of God.

This can be you.

I wasn't always like this. My transformation was actually pretty recent.

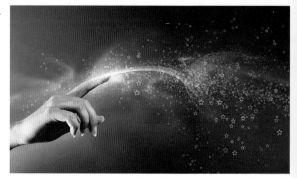

MY TRANSFORMATION

I almost died half a dozen times in my life because of stupid things I did... most of them lifestyle choices. I never drank alcohol, smoked, did recreational drugs or anything like that. I followed all the rules like a good citizen. But my life still came very close to ending numerous times. Why? Not because I played with guns or jumped out of airplanes. No, I had heart disease, liver disease, lung disease, I was hemorrhaging and had a list of medical problems longer than this book... all because I ate what I wanted: the modern American diet. For the first thirty years, I ate candy, hamburgers, florescent sodas, macaroni and cheese, pop tarts, toast, spaghetti, TV dinners, pastries, canned food, cheese, bread, milk, sugar, sugar, sugar and more sugar. I had cysts before I was even out of my teens. I couldn't drive more than a few minutes without stopping, opening the car door and coughing up a gob of mucus so I could breathe. People didn't call me Markus, they called me Mucus.

Like most people, the sad part is I really didn't know exactly what to do about it. It took me twenty years of experimenting, self discovery and research to figure it out. I tried every health fad there was.

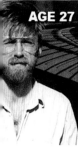 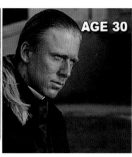 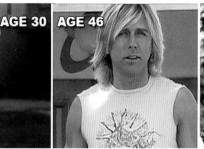 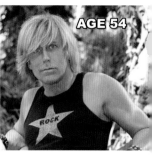

AGE 27 AGE 30 AGE 46 AGE 54

I became vegetarian, but still got sick. I tried every supplement on the market but still got sick. I became vegan. Still got sick. I tried it all. It wasn't until I finally had nothing left but the very basic fundamentals of life: air, water, sunshine, exercise, fruits, vegetables, love and the courage to listen to the quiet voice of truth (God/Universe), that it finally all made sense and a whole new world was opened to me.

It was like a door got opened, bright sunshine filled my face, angels sang and I stepped across the threshold from a world of dark illusion into a glorious new consciousness. Words can't describe the feeling of that moment. It all made sense. And how elegantly simple it all was! It was SO SIMPLE, a child could understand it. Any animal, plant or living being could understand it. It had nothing to do with knowledge or brains. It had to do with awareness of right and wrong.

Of only doing things that honor and appreciate life. I honor life. It blesses me in return with more life. By doing a few little sacrifices of not giving in to temptation (like comfort foods), we are rewarded with eternal health. Not only do our bodies become free of worldly burdens, but our souls - our very essence - are allowed to shine and express themselves and sing and dance with all the universe. We radiate a loving energy that blesses everything it touches. We become a beacon of light that heals others. We become givers of life instead of takers. And as a reward, we are given the ability to finally truly appreciate the mate we are with. To feel their skin in such a way you never knew possible. To have the gentle sound of their breath send waves of indescribable bliss through your being so strongly that every hair on your body stands on end. Imagine living life that way.

You can.

And it starts right now.

15

All it takes is a commitment from you that you will do whatever it takes. No turning back. For some it won't be easy because of addictions. This is like joining the police academy. There is a war going on and it takes total dedication and honor to stay true and win. The good news is: those who join DO WIN!!! Even those who join during the last days of their lives are glad they did, because they know it is the right thing to do. They go out with a free heart and a pain-free loving smile on their face.

I want to see a world where no one dies in a sterile hospital room any more. When we go out, it will be under a beautiful blue sky having an orgasm. People, …it's time to live !

It's never too late to be what you might have been.

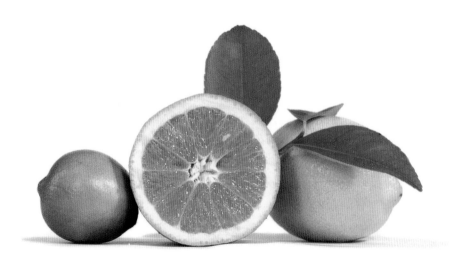

WHAT ABOUT GENETICS?
It's Never Too Late to Make it Right

This one really gets me going. Firstly, <u>you are NOT a helpless victim when it comes to genetics.</u> Most conditions - even genetically-based - are not as much genetic as inherited lifestyle and diet habits, because the body is adaptive. Even if you actually inherited defective genes, guess what, <u>DNA can be altered!</u> Nobel prizes have been awarded over these amazing discoveries. DNA proteins have been observed to adapt in as little as a few minutes sometimes to a new environment. Read the book "The Genie in Your Genes". Your genes and DNA can actually be radically altered by your thoughts and emotions, for better or worse.

Poor diets and toxic environment make the cells deficient and toxic when they are formed, and become worse with each formation, leading to illness. <u>Don't blame genetics.</u> Since DNA adapts, blame environmental chemicals, prescription drugs, negative emotions and unnatural diet choices. Genetic predisposition is not a pre-doomed fate.

Genes do affect our cells, but not nearly as much as people would like you to believe. Genes do not have the final say. You do. All you need to do for health is give your cells what they need and protect them from what they don't need. If all of your cells are healthy, you cannot be sick. Our bodies produce more than 10 million new cells every second, as we constantly rebuild our tissues. Old cells are constantly being replaced with new ones. If new cells are not built with proper raw materials, they will be unhealthy and weak.

<u>CHOICES make you, not inherited genetics</u>

Genetic damage can be repaired. Even when people say "nothing can be done about it". Amazing new discoveries are scientifically proving that almost anything is possible.

The proper emotional mindset is the foundation. Eliminating deficiency and toxic stuff, then allows the body to self-repair, and what many consider nothing short of "miracles" start to happen.

Your moment to moment choices determine whether your cells become healthy or get sick.

Don't Blame your Parents.
Although we inherit genes from our parents, how we maintain and care for our genes determines everything. Maybe you inherited a junker, but you can strip it down and rebuild it.

AVOID:

Sugar and too much sweet stuff, stress, noise, negativity, fear, distractions, processed food, baked goods, bread, pasta, wheat flour, milk,cheese, meat, eggs, fish, food preservatives, prescription drugs, anti-depressants, steroids, grilled, char-broiled, heated, cooked, fried or boiled foods radiation from X-rays, cell phones, plastic water bottles, environmental chemicals

It's not the cards we are dealt, but how we play the game. If you are born sick, make yourself healthy. Rebuild yourself into something new. The choice is YOURS. And your body will adapt. Stop blaming your illnesses on aging or faulty genes, rather than on its true cause. Maybe you are genetically predisposed to getting a certain condition, but proper lifestyle and nutrition will help determine if that condition will ever happen at all.

Let's compare you with a delicate wine glass. Your "genetic" disposition is that if you fall, you break, just like all the other wine glasses that fell. And over many years of use, your odds will increase of breaking. But what if you took really good care and treated yourself like a rare museum piece? You could go for CENTURIES without ever breaking. The choice is yours.
Heredity is secondary to environment and you control your environment.

"People often give up on their genetic predispositions, relieving themselves - at least in their own minds - of responsibility for their actions. They say 'There is nothing I can do, weight problems run in my family'(as they gulp down a burger, fries and large shake.)
It's bizarre that physicians put so much stock in the genetic origins of disease yet also inflict massive amounts of genetic damage with pharmaceutical chemicals and X-rays."

Dr. Ruza Bogdanovich

Watch what you say and how you feel. Words have unbelievable power. Most people say things in a way that increases stress and weakens the body's immune system. Words are powerful, they totally change the way we think and feel and research has conclusively shown that they actually change our DNA! Read the book "The Genie in Your Genes". Speak positively, not negatively, it can change your life.

If you are not well and keep doing what you have done in the past, you will continue to get worse. Forget the genetic thing. Take responsibility for your actions and health <u>right now</u> !

They must find it difficult...
Those who have taken authority as the truth,
Rather than truth as the authority."
G. Massey, Egyptologist

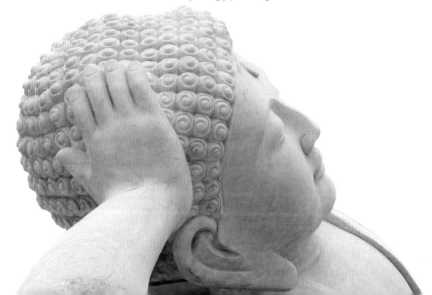

BACTERIA, VIRUSES AND CANCER
ARE NOT THE BAD GUYS

We all have cancer cells, salmonella, E-coli, candida, aids and parasites in our body. Every one of us. It is part of life. They are sitting there dormant, waiting to do their job. The first thing we need to realize is these AREN'T the bad guys. They are the sanitation workers of life. Their job is to eat up unhealthy weak and dying stuff. It is their job to return us to the earth so we can be recycled. Only the sick and dying are recycled. If our bodies are healthy and clean, there is nothing to recycle so they don't do anything. But if we eat sugary, pasty dead food that weakens our body, and consume meat which our body isn't designed to fully digest so it starts to rot and putrefy inside us, then our body becomes toxic and weak inside. These weak cells and parts of our body then become targets for the appropriate sanitation workers to come to action and eat those weak parts of us. It's our job then to keep all parts of our body clean and healthy.

The first signs are tiredness, mood swings, body odor, bad breath, bleeding gums, itching; yeast infections, foot fungus, etc.
The next sign is smelly gas and poop - that means something is rotting inside you. (That's right - clean people on a 100% raw food diet do not have body excretions that smell.) Think about it; what do you think that smell is? Something is DYING inside you! And dead stuff usually has bacteria, maggots, parasites, mold and fungus to help break it down, right? It's no different inside the human body. Like internal rust on a car, the rust will eventually spread to the main frame and body. Stop it while you can! Don't be a bag of rotting garbage.

Nature by its infinite wonderful design is set up in such a way that only the strong and fit survive. If the sick and weak kept reproducing, a species would eventually die off. Therefore it's mandatory that only the strong survive and nature's insurance for that is that each of us has a built-in self-destruct mechanism if we don't take care of ourselves.

Don't blame the cancer cells; they aren't the bad guys, they are only doing their job. Proof of this is the fact that cancer is not random or contagious. It only picks those who have some weakness in their body/mind/spirit. Be careful with not just what you eat, but also what you say (negative affirmations) and how you think (depression, anger, anxiety, sadness, resentment, fear, jealousy, hatred etc.) Your negativity can literally eat you up! Start looking at the bright side of things - your survival literally depends on it! Stop feeling sorry for yourself - that's negativity and by doing so you are killing yourself. Don't be a martyr. People only want happiness in their lives, not sob stories, so don't solicit pity from others, you're only pulling them down... and for what? So they can be miserable like you? Why don't you heal yourself and become a shining example to them of how amazing you really can be... trust me - I've been there - you'll get a lot more attention becoming an inspirational example for them to look up to. They need inspiration. They might not show it, but they need you to prove to them what's possible. They'll ask you how you did it and then you'll really be a hero. And you'll have a long healthy happy sexy vibrant life to boot.

I did the "feel sorry for myself" route. Nobody cared. Nobody paid attention. It made me slip deeper into depression. People started avoiding me and it made me sicker. I almost slipped away into nothingness and few would have noticed. Is that what you want? NO!!! There are too many things on this planet to enjoy. Too much beauty to soak in. Too many opportunities for love, beauty, sex and touching God. And you want to know the irony of how you get out of the slump? Get this... here it is, the big secret... (drum roll)...
Get rid of the rotting crap in your life: clean out your body, your mind your soul... and you start soaking in the beauty. Love everything in sight. Make love like there is no tomorrow. See God in everything everywhere. The secret is to stop dwelling on the negative bad stuff in your life (self pity) and just plain forget about it and GET ON WITH YOUR LIFE!!! Smell the roses!!!! Tell everyone you love them. Listen to beautiful music. Inspire yourself. Do whatever it takes to feel PEACE in your life.

Leave that stressful job and relationship. If you are too scared, read my pocketbook *Instructions for a New Life* and *The Prosperity Secret*. Make peace with yourself and everyone and everything. Only put things in your body, mind and spirit that are made by Nature - plant food that grows in nature, thoughts that make you feel good, and love. That's it. KEEP IT SIMPLE. Simplify your life to these basics and learn to breathe again! Life does not have to be complicated.

Is your glass half full or half empty? It's the same glass - but be careful which perspective you choose, because one answer will enliven you and the other will kill you. Same glass. The only difference is your choice of view. Your choice.

You are not a victim.

The choice is yours.

You have everything you need.

The choice is yours.

Start right now, this second!!!

OK, to sum up the last chapter: **You don't cure illness and disease by simply killing bacteria or taking magic herbs.** You stop feeding them (sugar, bread, meat, cheese, milk etc)... you starve them and usher them out the back door. If you eat what you are supposed to eat, most of these guests will pack up and leave. If you have an unwanted house guest, you don't kill them, you help them pack and show them the door.

This does not mean you will have a life of boring bland food. Quite the contrary. But we'll get into that later.

My point is: **health comes from getting rid of bad stuff, not simply adding some miracle stuff** to your regimen. That usually never works. You need to stop doing what's bad for you and clean out the mess inside first. Then you only put good, highly nutritious raw living enzyme-rich natural foods back in, along with lots of oxygen, sunlight and clean healthy water... and then you swish it all around with exercise and positive loving thoughts and energy.

Nobel prize winner Alexis Carrel was able to keep tissue cells alive indefinitely by supplying nutrients and more importantly washing away cellular excretions. In other words- keep yourself clean !!!

Lab rats lived twice as long when their food was cut in half.

It's not how much we eat. It's what we eat and more importantly CLEARING THE WASTE OUT that can really bring us vibrant results. The more cleaning out we do, the longer we live.

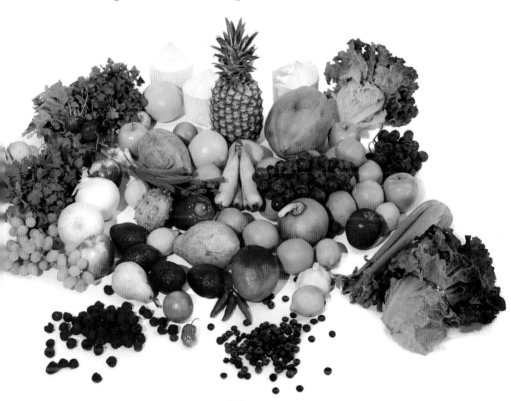

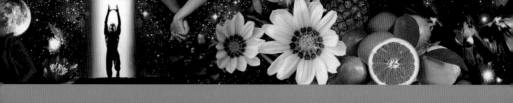

HERE WE GO

WHAT WE CAN LEARN FROM ANIMALS

OK. I'm just going to get right to it. Ready ?
I'll give away the secret in this very first sentence:

Don't cook your food.

This one statement can totally change your life.

Man is the only creature on the planet that cooks his food and the only creature that gets cancer, heart disease, diabetes, Multiple Sclerosis, leukemia, bla bla bla. The only animals that get those diseases are ones fed by man or eat garbage left over by man.

When you heat food above 118F, 45C it kills the enzymes and enzymes are what makes every bodily function work. Enzymes are necessary for life. Notice how tired you feel after eating cooked food. (Raw foodists don't have that.) When someone eats cooked food, their white blood cell count goes up because cooking alters the chemical structure of the food and the body doesn't recognize it, so it sends in the immune defenses to fight it. That's right: our body is fighting the very food we are eating!

That's why we get so tired... plus the fact that digesting food takes a LOT of energy (almost 2/3 of our energy goes to digesting food). The longest living people on the planet don't eat very much. The body doesn't really need a lot of food. Most people who have disease eat way too much and they eat dead lifeless garbage. We have strayed so far from nature it's sad.

People who stop eating processed cooked food notice their diseases start going away. They lose weight and find energy they never had before. Hmmm.

Look at animals in the wild. You CAN'T TELL HOW OLD THEY ARE. Once they reach full size, they look the same pretty much until they die. Ever wonder why?
Because they follow natural laws of living, eating and being. They eat things the way they are found in nature. They don't process food, grind it into flour and bake it. They don't saute it in pans with oil, or boil noodles or make crackers out of it.
They also don't suppress emotions. If they feel something, they do something about it. They don't whine about their problems to other animals and bore them with self-pity. They also don't drink alcohol or soft drinks... they don't smoke or sit around all day on a computer or watch TV. They don't party all night and drink beer and eat chips. What they DO is wander a lot, explore the world, get fresh air, sunlight, eat naturally, find a mate and make love whenever they feel like it. They rest when they're tired and get up with the sun. They play whenever possible. They don't need fancy material things.

"Does raw food include raw meat ?"

It would if you were a carnivore like dogs, cats, tigers and lions. But we are not designed that way. Carnivores have stomach acid ten times stronger than ours. That's why you see them swallowing whole animals without chewing very much - fur, feathers, bone - everything... GULP, down it goes. The stomach acid is so strong it can dissolve a whole animal. Humans can't do that. A carnivore's digestive tract is very short,

25

so the digesting contents can get out of the body as fast as possible before it becomes toxic. Humans have a very loooong digestive tract, where rotting flesh just putrefies, ferments and causes disease. Yes we are ABLE to eat meat and survive, but it is only a survival option in case we need it. It is not optimal for real health. Many animals only eat other animals when they have to... when there is nothing else. A brown bear is almost completely vegetarian. They eat mainly berries and leaves. By the way, one square inch of raw meat (like sushi) usually contains over 10,000 parasite eggs and larvae just waiting to hatch inside you.

Animals in the wild are protected from parasites by that super-strong stomach acid. Domestic animals are not so lucky because we feed them canned food, kibble and processed crap so their stomach acid is weaker and that's why they end up getting worms and parasites just like we do.

Diets high in animal foods turn kidneys to stone because the body needs lots of calcium to process the high levels of animal protein (plant protein doesn't do this). Animal products are the number one cause of diabetes because they contain saturated fat that clogs our cells and insulin receptors preventing insulin from allowing sugar to enter cells (insulin resistance).

Let this one fact inspire you more than anything: Cultures that eat the least amount of meat live the longest. Blue Zone people eat very little meat.

WHAT ABOUT PROTEIN ?

This has to be the most asked question of all. It's another great example of how brainwashed we all are. Protein is made from amino acids and almost EVERYTHING in nature has amino acids. The largest animals on the planet don't eat meat. Where do they get all that muscle from? What do elephants, rhinoceroses, buffalo, cows and horses eat? Mainly grass, leaves and fruit. Gorillas are five times stronger than humans. They have sharp canine teeth... but what do they eat? Leaves and fruit. They are vegetarians. If there was no protein in grass and leaves, horses would not exist. Pound for pound, molecule for molecule, there is more nutrition, more protein, more healing power and life force in plants, leaves, fruits, vegetables and seeds than anything else. The secret trick is to break apart the tough cellulose to release all that goodness, and THAT'S the difference between a cow and humans, and that's where most people screw up. Cooking isn't wise. Chewing it a few times and

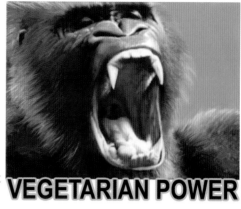

VEGETARIAN POWER

swallowing it doesn't do it. More on that in a minute.

But what about meat as a source of protein? Is it healthy?

The longest living animals on the planet are non-meat eaters.

The bodies of meat eaters full of corrosive ammonia. Meats are highly inflammatory (that's why meat eating animals don't live as long).

People don't get cancer from plant protein.

Meat vs. Plant protein: *THE CHINA STUDY*

"The China Study" is the largest, most comprehensive study ever done on this subject...
Cornell and Oxford University researched the effects of ingesting meat versus plant food on 650,000 people in Indonesia in 26 provinces over the course of 22 years. One group of people was fed meat while the other group was fed only plant foods. The group that was fed meat and animal protein developed cancer while the group that was fed raw plant foods stayed healthy. Then the foods were switched on them and the people who had cancer were fed raw plant foods and they got healthy again! The healthy group that was fed meat got cancer! This was replicated 50 times over the course of 22 years!!! See: TheChinaStudy.com.

It's important to know that the body makes protein from AMINO ACIDS. It cannot take animal protein and simply plug it into our cells. Our body has to break down meat into a liquid state (that's a LOT of work!), and then break it way down to basic amino acid molecules... then reassemble them into HUMAN form protein bonds that only a human body can use. This takes a lot of energy and time and is an inefficient way of getting protein. Add to that the fact that animal products (including dairy) are highly inflammatory and filled with hormones, antibiotics, steroids and raised on cheap, unhealthy animal feed. Even if the animal was raised organic, it's natural hormones are not meant for human use. A cow has hormones that make it grow fast to weigh thousands of pounds. If we eat this cow or drink its milk, it makes things in US grow fast, like cancer. Animal products are a foreign protein and foreign proteins are the base for most disease in the human body. Add to that the alien fast-growing hormones and you have a recipe for disaster. Consumption of strange indigestible proteins and runaway sugars that feed pathogens may be among the causes of most disease.

The protein in plants does not have uric acid or saturated fat to clog your arteries like meat does or IGF-1 animal growth hormone that causes cancer. The kidneys of the meat eater must work three times harder than the kidneys of the vegetarian.

I could go on and on.

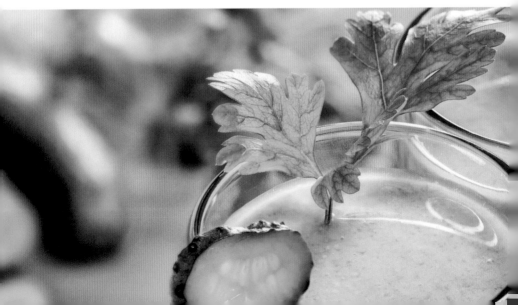

HEALTHY NON-MEAT SOURCES OF PROTEIN:

First, do NOT take whey protein. Whey is dairy.

Secondly, stop worrying about protein. It's a waste of energy. Where do horses, apes, elephants, buffalo and so on get their protein and muscles from? Grass and Greens. There is some serious power in that green stuff. Since we are lazy and don't CHEW our food like a horse or cow does, the best way for humans to get the most out of greens is to throw the stuff in a blender. BZZZT: instantly digested and all the cellulose broken apart for us. (Vitamix, Blendtec, and now the Markus blender are the best blenders). The wild chimpanzee diet is probably the closest thing to what we should be eating, and Victoria Boutenko wrote a book about it, "Green for Life". Basically, chimps eat mainly half fruit and half green stuff. They don't eat nuts but eat a few seeds and only eat roots when there is nothing else to eat (for us that would be carrots, beets, turnips, etc). SO, bottom line, you can get your protein from a blended drink of strawberries and kale, or banana and romaine lettuce, or mango and spinach and so on. (See blender ideas later in book).

That said, here is a list of stuff that's really high in protein...

CHLORELLA 62% amino acid content. This algae is considered one of the most complete foods on the planet: you can live off this stuff indefinitely. It has ALL the amino acids (a complete protein), more than any whole food on Earth, plus all kinds of minerals, enzymes, chlorophyll and pretty much everything else... Beta carotene (Vit A), C, E, K, B complex B1, B2, B6, B12, niacin, pantothenic acid, RNA, DNA, folic acid, biotin, choline, and inositol. Phosphorus, potassium, magnesium, germanium, sulfur, iron, calcium, manganese, copper, zinc, iodine, cobalt, and trace elements. It replicates so fast, it quadruples every twenty-four hours. (Amazing genetics). It also quadruples our friendly flora probiotics), making it one of the most potent growth factors available.

(Listen up bodybuilders). It boosts the immune system immensely (helps children grow and stay healthy), helps digestion, alkalizes, heals intestinal lining, helps remove chemicals, toxins and heavy metals from the body. It enhances health and muscle growth, increases the concentration of hemoglobin in red blood cells(for iron and oxygen), helps reduce cholesterol, and helps the liver to detox.

Best taken on an empty stomach at least 20 minutes before other food. Chlorella is in both my Protein and Green Formula

PINE NUTS (pignolia) contain more protein than any other nut or seed in the world. Native Americans and Russians used pine nut soup as a replacement for mothers milk. They are also high in healthy fats, dietary fiber, zinc, organic sulfur (MSM), iron and a great source of prostaglandins- a vital group of hormone-like substances derived from essential fatty acids that regulate body functions electrically. Prostaglandins are key to health, heart, hormones, fertility, cholesterol, eyes, anti-aging, inflammation and controlling disease. Pine nuts are a super rich food source and an awesome source of protein, fats, fiber and energy. Pine nuts are also a key ingredient in my protein formula.

SEA VEGETABLES (at least 50% protein), can compete head-to-head with animal proteins and are much more assimilable. Sea greens have more minerals than anything else on the planet. They are also the best source of iodine, needed for a healthy thyroid.

Examples: Dulse, Kelp, Kombu, Arame, Wakame, Irish Moss, Nori, Bladderwrack

Put in smoothies, soups, salads or make entire meals out of them. Eat every day. We have numerous recipes using Sea Moss in our cookbook.

PINE POLLEN & BEE POLLEN are some the best of all high protein foods

TOCOTRIENOLS (rice bran solubles) A good non-heavy protein powder that's great for smoothies. This is also the very best source of vitamin E.

QUINOA gluten-free Incan supergrain with complete protein from amino acids and complex carbohydrates. Soak and eat. Do not cook.

ACAI BERRY has almost an identical protein and amino acid profile as that of an egg.

DURIANS (pictured below) smell really bad but are worth it. They are a great source of protein; a favorite food of orangutans, elephants, tigers etc. They also have high levels of tryptophan (good for depression, insomnia) and raises brain serotonin levels (makes you feel good). You can get them in Asian markets. The frozen kind are not as smelly. Leave them in sink overnight to thaw. See my video at **DurianRecipe.com**

HEMP SEEDS (no this isn't the kind you smoke!) At 30 grams of protein per tablespoon, hemp seeds are a very popular source of protein in the health world. Hemp seeds contain all nine essential amino acids.

MESQUITE MEAL used as a staple food for centuries by desert dwellers. High protein, with good quantities of calcium, magnesium, potassium, iron and zinc, lots of amino acid lysine with a sweet rich molasses-like flavor and a hint of caramel. Blends well into smoothies..

FAVA BEAN (Broad bean) They have so much protein, they are called the meat of the poor. A mere 1/4 cup has 10 grams protein. Highly nutritious and full of many essential nutrients required by the body. One of the main foods around the world for 5000 years, especially the mediterranean Greeks and Romans. Fava beans are super high in L-dopa. a brain neurotransmitter that helps control hypertension. Fava beans help the body create HGH, the anti-aging natural growth hormone that also helps muscle growth. See my video at **FavaBeanRecipe.com**

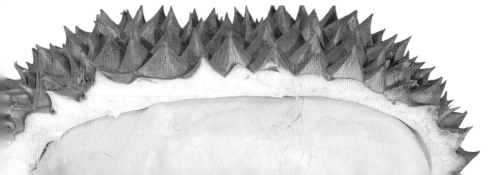

MORE PROTEIN:

Nettles
Seeds (soaked)
Nuts
OlivesGreen vegetables like spinach, watercress, arugula, kale, broccoli, brussel sprouts, collard greens and parsley
Grasses like wheatgrass, alfalfa, barley
Blue-green algae
Spirulina
Pumpkin seeds
Almonds
Brazil nuts (contain selenium)
Sprouted wild rice, sprouted grains & Sprouts of all types

Soak seeds, nuts and grains before eating to dissolve away the enzyme inhibitor coating (making them easier to digest). Overnight is best. Soak at least a few hours. Seeds are better than nuts. (Cashews are not nuts and don't need to be soaked) For busy people on the go who just don't have time, I have developed a super raw food protein powder, at MarkusProtein com

FASTING ACTUALLY HELPS: studies performed at Cornell University show that when a person fasts for 24 hours the body doesn't lose any protein, only fat. Bodybuilders who fast one day a week actually gain more muscle mass faster because the body is cleaner and more efficient.

Let's get started.

Firstly: you don't get healthy by simply adding something to your diet - it's what you take away that makes the big difference. If you have a rusty car, no amount of super fuel is going to make it run much better, unless you clean the rust away first. The cleaner the parts are, the better it will run. The same goes for your body. It's time for some serious spring cleaning.

CLEANSING
THE MOST IMPORTANT SECRET OF ALL

Nutrition is important, but it's the cleansing that
makes the difference - Paul Nison

When we rebuild an old junk car or house, we have to strip it down to its bare skeleton and scrape away every bit of rust and termites. Health does not start by popping some pills or health food. No. We have to strip our bodies down and clean out all the garbage and plaque from our cells that have been accumulating since we were born. Believe it or not, people are still carrying with them the residues of bad food and thoughts from childhood. Yes, our cells regenerate and replace, but the message is passed down through cell generations. Cells have memory.

Even people on a healthy raw living food diet need to cleanse, or else even they will end up with a health challenge of some kind. Why cleansing is so important, even for healthy raw foodists, is because the body needs to get rid of millions of dead cells every day, not just food. Dead cells are toxic and need to be removed quickly. About 100 pounds of dead cells are sent to our bowels every year. Without proper cleansing, fiber and colon cleansing, we accumulate more waste than our bodies can handle.

WHY ARE MANY RAW FOODISTS SO SKINNY ?
(AND HAVE GAS)

Remember, the answer is not simply "what to eat or take" but what to get rid of. Eating all the raw food in the world won't do much good if it doesn't ABSORB into your body. It needs to be clean to work right. You must clean out first... and continue doing so regularly. Not doing regular colonics or enemas is one of the biggest mistake raw foodists make. They need to cleanse just as much as everyone else. Why? Because when you clean house, you have massive amounts of garbage and unused stuff getting dumped out... so much it overfills your existing garbage cans. You need extra help to get rid of that garbage.

If you don't, this stuff will clog up your house and make it even uglier than before. In other words, a raw food diet makes your body detox. It pulls years and decades of toxic garbage from your cells and fills up all your "garbage cans"; your lymph system is overburdened, your liver and kidneys fill up suddenly with waste and your elimination system is overwhelmed from this mass exodus. If you don't send in more help to carry this stuff away, it will reabsorb into your bloodstream and make you more sick and toxic.

Secondly, raw foodist or not, most people's stomach acid is way too weak. In nature, many things are bitter, not sweet. Bitter stuff helps digestion, strengthen the liver and help create stomach acid, but most people only go for sweet stuff, often avoiding all bitter things totally.

Thirdly, the cellulose in raw vegetables is tough to digest - it requires a pH of 1-2, which no one has. Cellulose requires the enzyme cellulase to digest and that's one of the few enzymes that our pancreas doesn't create, it needs to come from outside sources. All raw fruits and vegetables contain cellulase, but many people switching to raw food don't actually eat a lot of living raw food, believe it or not (especially leafy greens), they eat raw chocolate, raw cheesecake made from cashews, raw coconut smoothies, lots of dehydrated crackers, cookies, cakes and desserts... lots of SUGAR (which weakens stomach acid and promotes parasites... and no cellulase enzyme... so when they DO eat greens... the food doesn't get properly digested and ends up fermenting, creating GAS.This undigested food also won't assimilate into the body, so they end up starving nutritionally and become skinny. Add to that other causes of low stomach acid like stress, lack of herbal vitamin C, zinc, B vitamins, lack of proper sleep, smoking stuff etc. This nutritional deficiency makes hair turn grey, robs energy and ages people. That's why there are grey haired, skinny wrinkly people who are shriveling up and think they are "healthy". The answer is to raise the stomach acid and blend more of the food you eat. Raw foodists who eat less sweets and more bittrer greens every day start getting normal weight back, lose wrinkles and even sometimes their grey hair goes dark again. More on that later.

Cleansing must be a regular thing, because even once we are clean (or think we are), we are constantly breathing in toxic air (100% of women tested had jet fuel in their breast milk), drinking water from toxic plastic water bottles (chlorine in drinking water scars our arteries and the plastic is a cancer causing estrogenic), eating food with who-knows-what in it, touching doorknobs and shaking hands with parasites on them, and also absorbing negative thoughts and energy from others. Even raw foodists "cheat" with food regularly. A little tiny thing here and there while traveling, a meal out with family or friends there. It all adds up. Cleansing must be regular. You can always tell who isn't doing enough cleansing when some raw foodists get sick or die like "normal" people... while others live way past 100.

OK. Let's start with common everyday foods we are addicted to and why they are destroying you.

MILK, CHEESE and DAIRY

(including cheese, yogurt, ice cream, sour cream, white salad dressings etc)

Be aware that ALL humans are lactose intolerant, just to different levels. Countries consuming the most milk products also have the highest rates of bone fractures, degenerating bone disease (like osteoporosis), heart disease, breast cancer, allergies, diabetes and multiple sclerosis. The United States consumes more dairy than the rest of the world put together and yet has the highest levels of osteoporosis and weak bones in the world.

Milk does NOT put calcium in our bones, it does the opposite: it PULLS calcium from our bones, making them weak, soft and brittle. Why? Dairy products are inflammatory to our body, which forces our body to normalize pH by pulling alkaline minerals from wherever it can get them, namely our bones, to neutralize the acids. This ironically leads to calcium deficiency. Cows' milk is not the same as human milk. The calcium in cows' milk or cheese is not the same as calcium from organic plant sources like leafy greens (that's where cows get their calcium!) Plant calcium absorbs into our system much easier.

35

Milk and cheese are among the leading causes of arthritis, constipation, allergies, asthma, colic, sinus issues, heart disease, ovarian problems, anemia, insulin-dependent diabetes, cataracts, obesity, congestion, lung problems and even cancer. These dairy products have been directly linked to heart attacks and strokes. When people are autopsied, they cut open the heart and all this white thick goo pours out... guess what it is? Calcium plaque! That's like trying to use cement instead of oil in your car's engine.

Dairy creates mucus which clogs up our intestines, lungs and reproductive systems, overloading them with slimy mucus that smothers our cells so they can't breathe. When white spots start appearing on different parts of the body, it means fat and mucus has spread throughout the respiratory and reproductive systems. Hormonal imbalances often result, including thyroid, pancreatic and gonad dysfunctions. This condition results in cysts and tumors, eventually leading to cancer, especially breast, colon and reproductive areas. All animal products lead to fat and cholesterol deposits in the arteries and heart, lining them with a white thick pasty "cement" made of inorganic calcium. (which is different than absorbable calcium from plants).

Nothing clogs up your intestines faster than cheese and dairy. You might as well be swallowing glue.

Cows' milk contains much higher levels of saturated fat than human milk, meaning cholesterol buildup and blood circulation problems in babies and adults. Animal fat is a leading cause in diabetes, including type1 childhood diabetes. The worst thing you can do to a baby is give it cows milk.

Milk, cheese and butter is one reason more women are dying today of heart problems and breast cancer than ever before from saturated fat and animal hormones. People have all kinds of calcium clogging up their bodies. Without adequate magnesium to process the calcium, it is useless. More on that in a minute.

If you think cheese isn't an addictive substance, try to stop eating it.

Pasteurizing milk (boiling at high temperature) kills the enzymes, so the milk cannot be properly digested. The pancreas can't replace these missing enzymes, so here comes diabetes.

Homogenizing milk makes fat particles so tiny that they go through the intestinal mucus, directly into the bloodstream where they become an alien substance (like hydrogenated oils or margarine) that the body doesn't know what to do with, so they accumulate in the arteries, joints, heart and other organs.

Pasteurized milk is dead food. Calves (baby cows) fed pasteurized milk die after eight weeks!

Even if you could drink cows' milk raw, you wouldn't want to. Most cows are sick and diseased. They are milked by a machine causing blood and pus to be in the milk. Do you want to drink blood and pus?

When a human drinks cows' milk, only half of the protein is used, the rest becomes foreign protein in the body... and foreign proteins are the number one cause of all disease in humans. This puts a serious strain on the kidneys. The kidneys of a meat eater or someone who drinks milk or eats cheese have to work three times harder than the kidneys of a vegetarian. They ultimately turn to stone. Cows' products are very hard on a baby, because the kidneys aren't even fully formed yet.

A twelve-year Harvard study of 72,000 people showed that those who drank the most milk (three or more glasses a day) had more bone fractures than those who drank very little. Where do cows and horses, goats and elephants get calcium? From grass. Greens have more nutrition than almost anything on the planet. The best way to make greens digestible for humans is to chew them really well or put them in a blender with some fruit. That makes all the nutrients instantly absorbable.

Another important factor is MAGNESIUM. Calcium cannot be absorbed or utilized by the body without magnesium, and almost everyone today is dangerously low in magnesium. As a matter of fact, people are SO low in magnesium, that the first thing paramedics do when someone has a heart attack, is inject magnesium.

SO, take 1 teaspoon of magnesium several times a day. I personally take a product called Natural Calm, which is Magnesium Citrate, a white powder, I just put it in some water. Magnesium malate is even better.

FORGET STORE-BOUGHT SOY, NUT & RICE MILK

The concept is good but they contain isolated cargeenan and too much sweetener. Beware. Soy, almond, rice milk etc have all been boiled to death and lack the vitamins and nutrients of fresh live ingredients. Make your own healthy milk. They are super easy to make.

KEFIR

Kefir is a fermented product that's formed when probiotics are added to goat or cow milk or fruit juice or sugar water. In the case of animal milk, it digests the milk and lactose sugars, leaving a biologically active substance that is considered healthy by some people. There are two kinds of kefir: milk kefir and water kefir. One needs milk and the other can live off fruit juice, coconut water or just plain sugar water. After a few days, the sugar is digested and only kefir remains. This is really good for the digestive system. You can make your own by adding kefir "grains" to either milk or fruit juice. I don't use the milk kind. The problem with animal milk, especially cow milk is it contains hormones that make a calf grow to be a thousand pounds very quickly. This growth hormone causes unnatural things to grow in humans (like cancer and other hormone-driven diseases). Almost all animals are injected with steroids and antibiotics which kill the beneficial probiotic gut flora in babies and humans and dramatically lower the immune system. It's safer to stick with plant based kefir. While we're on the subject, fermented foods in general are super healthy and highly recommended for a healthy life.

So here are some easy, super fast ways to make milk alternatives that are much better for you and your children than the fluids from a cow...

Five Easy "Milks" in Under 1 Minute

You can even mix these together if you want

Banana Milk

(in blender)

1 frozen banana
1 cup water
optional: vanilla, cinammon, pinch of sea salt

Cashew Milk

(in blender)

1 1/2 cup cashews (better if soaked for 1 hr)
1 cup water
2 tablespoons Maple Syrup

Hemp Seed Milk

(in blender)

1 cup hemp seeds
2 cups water
Hemp seeds are VERY high in protein, B vitamins, calcium, iron

Almond Butter Milk

(in blender)

2 tablespoons of raw almond butter
2 cups water
a tiny pinch of sea salt
and a dab of raw honey or Maple Syrup (optional)

Coconut Milk

(in blender)

coconut water (the liquid from young thai coconuts)
some kind of **dark leafy greens (kale, spinach** etc)

note: don't use "coconut milk" from stores. It is boiled and highly processed

STAY AWAY FROM BREAD AND ANYTHING MADE WITH BAKED FLOUR

(Pasta, cereal, cookies, crackers, pizza, bagels, pastries, cakes, pies, muffins, pancakes, etc.) This is what almost killed me.

Aside from animal products, these foods are one of the major causes of illness in today's society. They are not found in nature.

BREAD is highly mucus-forming in the body. It's addictive and aging. Don't touch it. It's baked (heated), meaning all the life has been killed. It has almost no nutritional value. It turns into sugar in the body, which feeds parasites, bacteria, yeast, fungus, cancer and diabetes. It contains gluten, a very sticky substance that gums up your insides like glue paste and could lead to Inflammatory Bowel Disease, where ulcers eat holes in the intestines and you start bleeding when going to the bathroom. It contains an indigestible protein called gliadin, which is very tiny, so it gets easily absorbed into the bloodstream. Since the body doesn't know what this is, it causes all kind of problems with the immune system. It makes you tired and ultimately sick. It sticks to your teeth, causing tooth decay. Baked grains like wheat (especially when combined with dairy, butter and meat) may be causing over 100,000 early deaths per month in the USA alone.

The mucus formed from bread clogs your sinuses, lungs, liver, gallbladder, intestines and reproductive organs. There is no bread in nature. If you want to finally be rid of mucus, allergies, asthma, immune problems etc, stay away from wheat, bread and anything made with flour. Do you actually think you're going to build healthy cells from bread, cereal and pasta?

A university test was done where rats were fed nothing but "human food"... bread, sugar, eggs, milk, beef, potatoes, oranges, apples, bananas and coffee. The rats got diseases and didn't last long. If it can't keep rats alive... maybe you should think about this.

RICE?

Did you know Asia has the same rates of diabetes as the United States? A big reason is they are eating more meat and saturated fat, which is the biggest cause of diabetes. Meat and dairy spikes insulin TWICE as high as sugar! What makes it worse, is when it's mixed with starches and carbs like rice, the problem triples. Rice by itself isn't that bad, but when mixed with animal fat- watch out! The habit of mixing meat and potatoes or rice and fish is a dangerous one. Brown rice is better than white rice, but again, it's a cooked food, which is not as optimal for health as raw fresh plant food. It's not a "bad" food, and I have rice once in a while, but if you're trying to heal from something or do a serious cleanse, hold off on rice until later. There is a black rice called wild rice which can be eaten raw if soaked overnight. There are a variety of recipes out there.

GRAINS?

They require more work to digest than fruit which is why the body often gets tired afterwards. Most grains are so tough, they need to be cooked, which, like rice, make them less optimal for health and nutrition as fresh fruit, greens and veggies. Whole grains are best. You can't eat all grains raw, so save your cooked grains till after you are healed. Obviously steel cut oats prepared in hot (non-boiling) water is much better then oat bread. Try to never eat bread. There are some grains that CAN be eaten raw by soaking overnight like quinoa, millet, buckwheat, amaranth which are easier to digest. Oats and barley are ok also, but much denser (remember we are trying not to cook, only soak) Barley grass and sprouts are actually really good for you and super high in nutrients. It's in my green formula.

SUGAR IS POISON

This is not referring to whole or blended sweet fruit, but refined sugar. It's one of the most addictive and destructive foods on the planet. The only difference between cocaine and sugar is the time each takes to kill you. Next to cigarettes and stress, sugar is the fastest thing to age you. Sugar is rocket fuel for disease, viruses, bacteria, parasites, fungus, mold, yeast and anything that grows... including cancer cells.

Sugar water is what they use in labs to grow viruses when they study disease. Sugar turns into fat in our bodies. It demineralizes your body, pulls calcium from your bones, damages your immune system, leads to heart disease, high blood pressure, diabetes, arthritis, throws off your hormones, fries your pancreas and clogs your arteries because unused glucose becomes saturated fat and cholesterol, which is stored in your arteries, leading to high blood pressure and clots. Even worse, here's the scariest part: it cross-links proteins and causes your skin to wrinkle ! *GASP*

Forget cancer - egad - wrinkles are what people really fear! Want less wrinkles? Eat less sugar. It causes inflammation in every cell in the body. If you eat anything sweet (including honey, agave, anything super sweet), it's advisable to add cinnamon, which lessens the impact of sugar on the body by smoothing out blood glucose (sugar) levels.

OK, I covered the main basic addictive bad food stuff that hurts people… sugar, cheese, bread and especially meat and animal products. Many people find it's not too hard to become vegetarian, but it's real tough trying to lose the refined carbs. I know what a battle it is to try to not eat bread, cheese and sugar... but trust me, it's worth it.

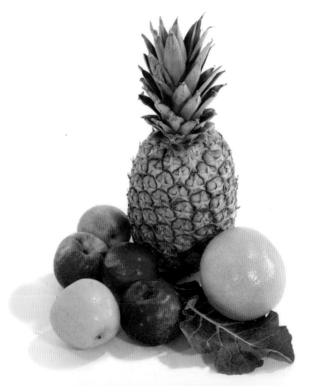

THE TRANSITION

SET YOUR OWN SPEED

Don't go into this reluctantly. That makes your stomach sour and defeats your willpower to succeed. You need to go into this WANTING to do this. If you only knew how amazing you will feel, you would jump in eagerly with both feet running. Be excited. have sunlight in your heart. Throw out all the darkness, doom and gloom in your life. You are creating a new you. You will shine. Imagine never being sick again. All you have to do is claim it. Something inside you needs to say "the future starts right now!". We're waiting for you at the other end my friend, and there is a party going on here. Come on over and celebrate! Don't look back and say "I should have done this years ago!" The main thing is to start walking in the right direction.

Go at your own pace.

Some people make the switch and go 100% overnight.
Some people have a hard time saying goodbye to bread, cheese, milk and meat, so they move to almond milk and veggie-burgers. They might feel a sense of accomplishment but not be completely healthy... but if that's what it takes to move in the right direction at a speed they are comfortable with... at least they are moving.

Some people go 100% raw and freak out a week later. They run back to their comfort foods, get sick again, then make another lunge at health and raw living. They go two steps forward, one step back. But at least they too, are moving.

Some people go all the way but stay in the comfort zone (this is most "raw" foodists). They go for all the sweet stuff, deserts and raw comfort foods. They practically live completely on raw chocolate, raw "cheesecake", raw cereal, raw ice cream, raw crackers, raw desserts, raw fruit smoothies, raw nut mixes... do you see what's happening here? They might have an occasional token salad or green juice... but they are basically still sugar/carbaholics. Sure, all that stuff wasn't heated. Yes, the enzymes are still intact. Yes, it's made with all natural raw ingredients. But they are not live foods anymore. Once something is liquified in a blender or food processor, all the cells are broken open and the life force is released. Moisture oxidizes, so within about 30 minutes, it's not vital anymore. It's just a sweet-tasting pile of minerals. Remember almost half of the diet should be fresh greens and most raw foodists eat nowhere near that. When tested, it was found that most of these people had almost no stomach acid at all! Bitter greens are necessary for proper digestion and a healthy liver, resulting in more energy, vitality, youth and nutrient assimilation.

BUT I must say this. Most of those people don't get sick much anymore. They are light years ahead of the rest of the country. And if they are open and enlightened to doing what's right, they will naturally gravitate to the next step.

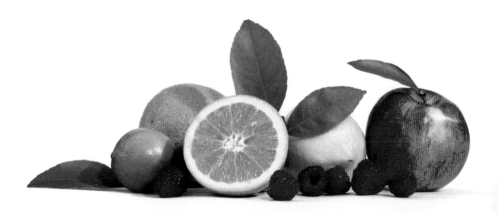

The ultimate goal is to eat minimal amounts of food. The longest living people don't waste their time eating or preparing food. They are busy LIVING. They are enjoying the world, each other and nature. They feel the wind and sun. And they eat very simply. Half fruit. Half greens. And a tiny bit of miscellaneous fun stuff... an egg now and then or a small fish or some nuts or roots, maybe even some raw milk from a goat. Most of all, they are care-free. They don't think too much about when their next meal is or where they are going to get it. Even if it's the next day or several days away, they don't care, because they know a human being can go months on nothing but water or juice. The healthier and cleaner we are, the more nutrition we can utilize from a single piece of fruit. It's like going 200 miles on a single gallon of gas.

The first step is knowing what <u>NOT</u> to do.

Avoid: sugar, bread, meat, cheese, milk, cream, butter, ice cream, eggs, fish, sodas, bread and anything made with flour - cereal, pasta, crackers, cake, pies, cookies, bagels, pitas, wraps, muffins - popcorn, energy bars, white rice, and of course cooked food - including steamed, sauteed, fried, boiled, baked - all commercial candy and chocolate, coffee, chips, and all processed food.

Stop smoking.
Stop drinking alcohol.
Stop drinking coffee.
Distance yourself from sources of stress.
Get rid of burdens, debt and anything negative.
Find a purpose.

Can you do this?

Do you want to live?
Do you want to be sexy and young again?

The choice is yours.

45

Once you are past the threshold, it's clear sailing. I know. Right now your mind is scared. Your addicted body is scared, craving what it knows, afraid to step into the unknown.

Trust me. You will never want to go back. This is like going from the dark ages to the supersonic age where people fly through the air. Come on. I'll give you something new to be addicted to... unlimited health and happiness. No more disease. No more being tired, overweight and depressed. Love and sex like you've never experienced before. Enlightenment beyond your wildest dreams.

There are some transitional foods you can eat to help you cross over.

Just be aware, soy cheese is not better; it's just as dead and worthless as dairy cheese and twice as high in cancer-causing IGF-1. Soy cheese does not grow in nature. It gums up our insides. Use hemp, almond, banana, cashew or sesame milk and cheese made with something like cashews, which, by the way, you can easily make yourself. These are much better and fresher than anything that's been sitting on a store shelf and was made five months ago. All kinds of recipes are in the uncookbook at **HealthyCookbook.com**

When you grind, juice or blend something, you are breaking it apart and killing it. It's nutritional vitality will only last a day or two. So it's best that you make as much of your food for yourself as possible. It's not that hard, it's a lot cheaper and you will feel much better, plus have a sense of satisfaction and accomplishment. (note: nutritional value can be preserved for a long time, even years, if moisture is removed immediately, as in powdering, …I'll explain later in this book) But lets keep things simple for now. Eat whole fresh juicy foods as much as possible. Blending, grinding and chopping is ok, but you should eat it right away.

You know what's amazing? The moment I started making my own healthy food, unhealthy friends that came over would always make their way into the kitchen and say "can I try that?". It was then that I realized how even what seemed like the last people on earth to want to change actually deep down inside were hoping to find something better and healthier in life. They were all amazed how GOOD everything tasted. My raw chocolate was always an instant hit. Wow, this isn't carrot-sticks and celery. Chocolate that's good for you and helps you lose weight? No heating or baking? Simply grind, mix with coconut oil and put in the freezer? It's really that easy? YES!

By the time I showed them how to make raw chocolate ice cream in 90 seconds with nothing but frozen bananas, cacao powder and a bit of vanilla, they were always hooked.
Within a month, most of them were doing colonics or enemas and calling me how much more energy and life-force they had.

WHAT ABOUT DEHYDRATED FOOD?

A lot of raw foodists get caught up eating lots of dehydrated food because it has those familiar hard and crunchy textures, or it's doughy... like bread. Dehydrated items should be considered transitional foods or travel snacks or occasional fun foods. But as fun as that stuff is, your main diet should be juicy fresh fruits and vegetables.

Dehydrators are machines that warm food no higher than 115 degrees F (45C) so the enzymes don't get killed. This could be compared to seeds and fruit falling to the ground in nature and the sun baking them until all the moisture is gone (dried fruit). Dehydrated foods taste good, but have no moisture. Many raw foodists make raw "bread" with dehydrators, or raw food energy bars, or raw burgers or cookies or macaroons etc. I ate a lot of these kinds of foods at first because they were very addictive.

Dehydrated foods are very dense though and suck moisture from your body. They require considerable energy to digest and might weaken your stomach acid. Again- they are great snacks and travel food, but it's always best to eat wet, moist fresh fruit and vegetables straight from the Earth, because we are wet, moist beings.

HOW AND WHY TO EAT

The next time you eat something, pay attention to how you eat, especially how you chew. I'll bet you chew only a bit until the texture of the food is lost and then you swallow... looking forward to that new virgin mouthful of new fresh crunchy texture... you like the feeling of it on your tongue, the way the hard goo feels crunching between your tongue and teeth... and when that fresh new sensation is gone, you swallow looking forward to the next fresh bite... right? Now pay attention to what you're swallowing. How big are the pieces? How digested are they really? Has anyone told you that your food needs to be fully liquified into a paste before swallowing? What makes you think your stomach is going to dissolve those un-chewed chunks? Where did you learn or assume that? Do you have any idea what you are asking of your stomach and digestive system? Are you starting to get an idea as to why you might be so tired and bloated after eating? Or why you aren't getting a lot of energy out of your food?

Food is supposed to be fuel. Most people eat for the wrong reasons nowadays in the modern world. They eat for stimulation. They want to feel that salty or sugary taste on their tongue, and that crunchy texture... or that hot spicy stuff mixed with sugar and they love the feel of the deep-fried crust with the gooey inside. They don't care what nutrition it has, as long as it makes them feel good, gives them energy and keeps them alive for another five hours. Am I right? It's all about temporary stimulation. Something in the back of their mind knows it's not really that healthy, but hey, what is one more plate of fried potatoes going to do? Surely this one meal isn't going to make any difference...

Unfortunately, it does. Every molecule you take in is either going to move you towards health or disease. There is no neutrality. Every bite in the wrong direction takes you that much further from health, and feeds disease... which you might not know is even happening until it's too late. Don't wait for that to happen. Start on the right path right now. It's not as bad and boring as you think. That's a misconception.
We are supposed to eat to give ourselves fuel, so that we can carry out

our dreams. Any food consumption beyond what we actually need is not just gluttony, it is bad for us, no matter how healthy the food is. Why? Because if our body doesn't need it, it goes to waste and starts to rot or turns to fat. It doesn't all simply poop out the next day. It waits around and clogs up our liver, blood, brain and organs, making us tired and lethargic. We think slower, move slower and feel slightly guilty, a negative emotion that attracts more negative energy into our lives. The less we carry around, the lighter we are, the lighter we feel, the less we attract heavy stuff into our lives. Want to be care-free? Eat light! Travel light.

The first thing we have to learn is that we don't need a lot of food to live healthily. Very very little. It's not how much you eat- what matters is how much you assimilate. And food must be fully digested to assimilate into your system and be useable.

CHEW YOUR FOOD!

Secondly, we need to relearn how to use our mouths. Until now, eating has just been about tasting the sugar, salt and food texture, but we didn't care much about actual digestion and health, so we half-chewed our food and swallowed. Everything we put in our mouth needs to be chewed until it is a creamy liquid, no chunks. Our stomach doesn't have any teeth and those chunks will go through you half-digested. Chewing your food until it is liquid goo increases how much benefit you get out of your food by as much as five times! This alone will increase your energy, keep you from being so tired after eating, getting gas, or getting sick, and even help you gain muscle more if you're working out or trying to gain weight.

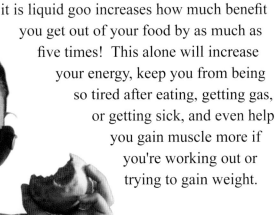

THINGS YOU'LL NEED

If you don't already have these, get them. You will need them.

A VEGETABLE JUICER

like the L'Equip (about $100).

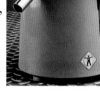

This extracts all the pulp and gives you only pure vegetable juice. This is what you use during juice fasting and serious healing/cleansing. Do not juice fruit because it concentrates sugar too much, only juice greens and vegetables. After this, you move on to blending where nothing is extracted, but everything is liquified.
For this you need...

A HEAVY DUTY BLENDER

like the **Vitamix** (pictured) or the one I have created- a blender so powerful it can liquify almost anything, but keeps the fiber and everything.<u>This is the most used and valuable piece of equipment I have</u>. It is so versatile it's amazing. I make everything from smoothies to pates to raw ice cream with it.

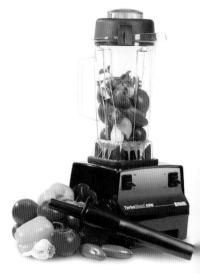

It cleans easy and will liquify any fruit and vegetable in seconds, making nutrients easy to assimilate in the body and saving digestive energy so that energy can be put towards healing instead. **If you only get ONE device- this is the one**!!!
(the Markus blender soon available at MarkusProducts.com)

Again... if you can only afford one device, get the super blender. Don't skimp and get a cheapie like a Ninja or Nutibullet. Your life depends on it.

Do I need a Vitamix? Is a normal blender OK ?

The Vitamix and Markus blenders do what a normal blender can't: it liquifies everything 100%. If you put fruit and vegetables in a normal blender, you'll have lots of small chunks and bits of fiber in there, which will probably end up being undigested food particles. Even if you are able to digest it all, it's extra work and strain on your body. Nothing compares to a Vitamix. I use it to pulverize branches and sticks to make herbal powders (after the vitamix breaks the herb branches down, I then use a coffee grinder and a sieve to make a really fine powder)

If you're absolutely broke and have no choice, then a normal blender is better than nothing. Don't let that be an excuse for not being healthy. I am working on developing a more affordable high-powered blender. Keep checking MarkusProducts.com for new stuff.

A general rule is- only use the juicer when you are sick or doing a cleanse, and the Vitamix pretty much all the time for the rest of your life, along with eating raw whole foods of course

Once you have a juicer and a blender, you are set. You might as well disconnect the power to your oven and stove. Some people use their oven to store pots and pans, and their stove as an area for sprouting. I keep one hot plate available to make tea.

AREN'T RAW FOODS EXPENSIVE ?

I hear things like this all the time: "I want to be healthy, but can't afford it", "organic food costs too much", bla bla bla. Yes, the first time people buy things at a Whole Foods Market, they get sticker shock. If that's the only place you buy food, yes it will cost more than normal grocery stores. Thinking you can't eat raw just because you have no money is a joke.

Check out what 36 dollars and 22 cents bought at the local Asian market... (!)

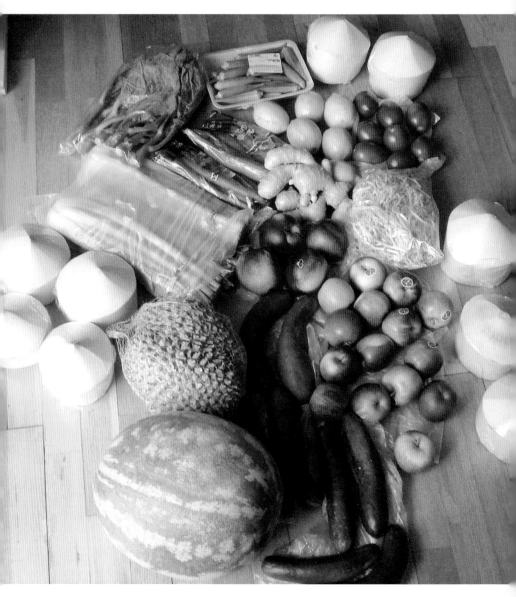

Ok, so it wasn't organic, but its still better than junk food. By the way, soaking fruits and veggies in water with 99 cent hydrogen peroxide in it neutalizes most pesticides. There was a period where I didn't make any money at all for almost two years, and I was still eating raw. There are no excuses.

What's the most important thing in your life? I would like to think the answer is BEING ALIVE, HAPPY and HEALTHY. The medical industry is a TRILLION dollar industry. Over one million people died last year in hospitals. Do you know what a kidney dialysis machine costs? More than your mortgage. How much do you spend every year on medication, doctor visits, dentists, chiropractors, over the counter crap like pain killers, steroids, cortisone, cough medicine, sleeping pills, stimulants, stress pills, skin creams, hemorrhoid creams, wrinkle creams, lotions, vitamin pills, Viagra, hormone pills, decongestants, stuff for itching, stuff for sore aching joints, impotence, incontinence, things to help you remember, keep you awake... and how about all that crap you buy for the gym like whey and soy protein powder, energy boosters, "get-big-quick" muscle crap, or magic weight-loss products? Seriously. How much do you spend? Look at that list again. Even if you are a vegetarian and think you are healthy... I know you still have health issues and spend money trying to heal. How much do you spend on soy cheese, soy milk, soy burgers, soy wieners, cereals, breads, pasta, cookies, crackers and other dead crap? Again- isolated soy protein is twice as high in cancer-causing IGF-1 as meat. Vegetarians are some of the unhealthiest people, who think they are "better" than others. If you want soy, eat soy beans, not processed crap.

What if you didn't need ANY of that stuff listed above? What if you never need a decongestant, pain killer, cough medicine or doctor visit ever again? What if your diseases went away and you never got sick again? What if you never got tired again and you had more energy and the hormones of a teenager, so much so that you were horny all the time? What would that be worth to you?

Now can you honestly tell me that organic fruits and vegetables are too expensive?

Many of you have medical insurance. How much do you pay per year for that?

Folks, I have a message for you...

THIS *IS* YOUR MEDICAL INSURANCE!!!

OK, I know some of you are really hard up financially and think you really can't afford it. This does NOT mean you can't be healthy. The healthiest, longest living people in the world live in "third world" countries like Pakistan, Africa and places in South America... and they barely eat much. They don't have cars, television, air conditioning, computers, internet, and they live in huts. They have much less money than you do, so if they can do it, so can you. I don't want to hear any excuses.

Right outside your window is stuff growing that is one hundred times more nutritious than anything you can find in a grocery store. They are more powerful than even organic food. They are starting to be sold in high-end health food stores. They are used to cure illness, disease and cancer. They are some of the most powerful liver cleansers known. They have lots of protein, antioxidants and powerful healing compounds. And they are FREE. They are weeds: Dandelion, Chicory, Mallow, Plantain, Chickweed, Yellowdock, and hundreds more. Every area in the world, no matter where you live, has weeds that can help you. For example, grass. Go to any gym or health bar and they sell wheatgrass juice for two dollars an ounce, whereas you could just go outside, grab a handful of grass and simply put it in your blender with some water. How much did that cost? As long as you didn't spray poisons on your yard, you have a treasure trove of healthy stuff growing wild and free around you. It is God's gift to the world. They sell dandelion greens at the local health food grocery store for four dollars a pound! I know the thought of eating "weeds" might seem strange, yet it shouldn't, because only modern society has labeled them that. That's someone's twisted, prejudiced opinion, no different than judging someone by the color of their skin or income level. Purslane, for example is considered a weed in America, but in the rest of the world, it's a vegetable. It's really good for you, it grows like crazy and it's FREE. Dandelion flowers have more lecithin than anything else on earth, even soy. You can live off nothing but dandelions if you wanted. Wild plants and herbs have over one hundred times the nutritional power of anything raised by man. Vegetables grown on a farm are raised in soil that's been used so much, year after year, probably for generations, that there is very little mineral content left. Also, these plants get watered every day and they know they will get watered every day, so their root system is very shallow and weak, maybe a few feet at best. Wild plants on the other hand might not get rain or water for months, sometimes even longer, so they grow very deep roots. Some weeds grow roots as deep as 100 feet or more! And that is through deep soil that's never been used. They go through layers and layers of mineral-rich earth and become super-rich with all the goodness available to them. Wild plants are survivors. They have a fighting spirit. They are not pampered, soft, wimpy and anemic like that grocery store fluff. Eat a survivor and you become a survivor.

There is so much wonderful nutritious food growing out there for free, all you have to do is go out there and grab it. Right across the street from me is a bunch of palm trees. The guy who owns the property just has them there for decoration. In the fall there are massive amounts of berries hanging from them that taste so sweet you would swear they were dipped in honey. They are Saw Palmetto berries. That's right, they enhance hormone production in men and are the world's best substance for prostate health. These berries are the number one ingredient in all medications and formulas sold at health food stores for prostate enlargement/cancer. Bodybuilders use Saw Palmetto to help boost their size production. Middle-aged men use it to boost their sex. And it's growing for free right outside my door. My friend Matt and I fill bags and bags with it.

There are so many houses in this neighborhood with fruit trees laden with fruit that nobody ever uses. The branches are so heavy with fruit, they touch the ground. All that beautiful fruit just going to waste! All over town, lemons, oranges, avocados, dates, persimmons, apples, grapefruit, ginkgo, olives, grapes, pears, peaches, currants, berries, nuts... a total feast. All you have to do is go ask permission to take some. And even if you paid them, it would be much less than any grocery store would charge. Did you know pine trees are edible?

My house has decorative **rosemary** plants growing all over the place. Rosemary is one of nature's finest antioxidants, specific for memory, brain function, stress, nerves and tension. Rosemary is rich in highly absorbable calcium and is used to fight breast cancer. I grab a handful every time I go from by backyard studio to the house.

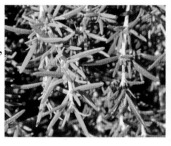

My front yard has numerous decorative **sage** bushes. Sage helps digest greasy fats, increases estrogen to treat menopausal sweats, keeps the stomach, intestines, kidneys, liver, spleen, and sexual organs healthy, encourages hair growth, increases circulation and relieves headaches, breaks fevers, and helps reduce respiratory congestion and cold symptoms. Simply chewing on sage cleans teeth and strengthens gum tissue.

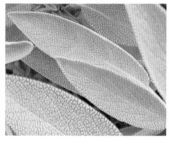

Those **dandelions** are God's gift to us. They are a worldwide super food and natural medicine. A great source of the antioxidant Vitamins A and E, B complex, C, D, calcium, iron, manganese, magnesium, phosphorus, potassium, sulfur, silicon, and phytoestrogens. It's used as a cancer treatment, a liver stimulant and tonic, to alkalinize the blood, to increase digestive acid levels, to lower cholesterol, as a diuretic, to cleanse the blood, as a lymphatic tonic, to improve circulation, as a mild laxative, and as a pain reliever. Dandelions help the entire digestive system. Dandelion roots are rich in minerals and trace minerals for bone, cartilage, tendon and ligament formation. Dandelions are blood cleansers, and remove acids from the blood. They are all the rage in health food stores now. Go outside and pick and grow your own! Every part of the dandelion plant is useful and edible; the roots, leaves, stem and flower (just not the fluffy part, that's for making wishes).

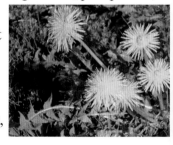

I planted some Aloe Vera in my yard a few years ago. It's grown into a huge patch. Every morning I go out and get some to put in my blender.

ALOE VERA

Aloe is one of the most amazing miracle food plants on the planet. It's so fantastic, it's like aliens put it here. It lasts forever and stores for months. Cut it and it <u>heals itself</u>! It's a smart plant; it can tell the difference between normal cells (which it stimulates), and bad stuff like viruses, cancer, leukemia or HIV, which it stops from spreading. It's used in AIDS treatment. It's antiviral, antibacterial, good for treating candida, parasites, fatigue syndromes, fibromyalgia, allergies, arthritis, and skin conditions like eczema and psoriasis. Aloe eliminates toxic wastes, has EFAs and is a powerful anti-inflammatory that helps the stomach and assists in cleaning the colon. Aloe helps every part of the body cleanse itself. It's especially great for the digestive system for conditions like indigestion, acid reflux, IBS, colitis, Crohn's disease and ulcers (reduces ulcers by 80%!). Aloe reduces cholesterol and triglycerides, helps metabolize fat and is great for... oh where do I start... adult diabetes, angina, blood sugar, cholesterol, acne, AIDS, allergies, anemia, arteries, arthritis, athletes foot, bad breath, baldness, bladder infections, bronchitis, bruises, burns, bursitis, cancer, candida, cataracts, cold sores, colic, colitis, constipation, cuts, cystitis... Aloe has all kinds of natural steroids, antibiotics, amino acids, minerals, enzymes and stuff we haven't even discovered yet. Put it on your skin and it soaks right through into your body and blood stream, going right to work. Speaking of SKIN, aloe is a miracle skin treatment; it's rich in organic silica and helps make strong cell and artery walls, mucous membranes, and the connective tissues of bones and cartilage, while healing skin cancers, hemorrhoids and varicose veins. It stimulates lymph movement and even has aspirin-like salicylic acid. Check out the video I did at **AloeCactus.com**, where I make an Aloe-Cactus drink, one of the most powerful drinks possible.

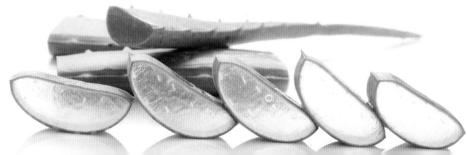

GRASS

Sure, go ahead, make fun of it. Snicker. Sweat uncomfortably at the
thought. But green grasses are the only plants on Earth that can give
sole nutritional support to an animal throughout life. They help with
high blood pressure, diabetes, gastritis, ulcers, liver disease, asthma,
eczema, hemorrhoids, skin infections, anemia, constipation, body odor,
bleeding gums, burns, even cancer. A good source of Vit K for blood
clotting. Good for bone strength and varicose veins. It's what horses eat
to become thoroughbreds. It's what elephants eat to become the biggest
land animals on the planet. All we have to do to break open the tough
cellulose structure to get to its benefits is juice or blend it. Personally, hate
wheatgrass and I believe it concentrates the sugars too much. I just throw
a handful of grass in the Vitamix so that I get the fiber, and it doesn't have
any taste. People, there are NO excuses. Nature is everywhere. It's all
around us. **And best of all, it's all FREE**!!!!

I created an amazing 480 page book on how to live on wild neighborhood
plants. It could change the way you look at the world around you..

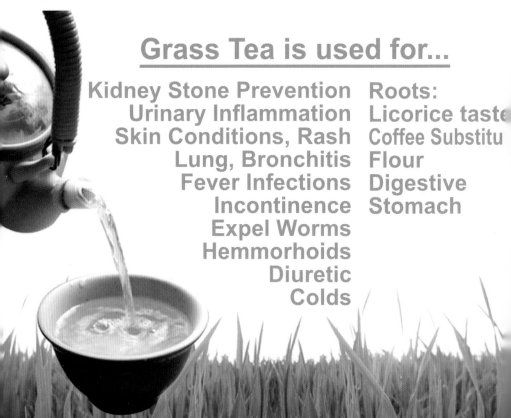

Grass Tea is used for...

Kidney Stone Prevention	Roots:
Urinary Inflammation	Licorice taste
Skin Conditions, Rash	Coffee Substitu
Lung, Bronchitis	Flour
Fever Infections	Digestive
Incontinence	Stomach
Expel Worms	
Hemmorhoids	
Diuretic	
Colds	

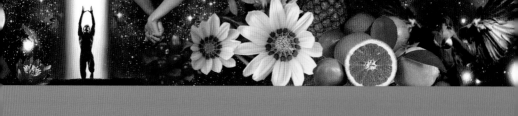

THE SHOPPING LIST

OFF WE GO TO THE GROCERY STORE

No, you can't stop and get some cheese tots and beer on the way.

Actually stuff from a farmers' market is fresher than groceries, or even better than that, grow your own stuff.

One of the biggest ruts people get into, even raw foodists, is that they eat the same foods over and over and over. Every time they go to the grocery store, they buy the same stuff. (Usually the stuff that tastes good to them). They get what they LIKE, not necessarily what they NEED. And guess what? They end up having deficiencies. Even if what they bought was super-nutritious, they would still develop deficiencies, because romaine lettuce has different nutrients in it than kale or collard greens or cabbage. They are made up of different things - that's what makes them different (duh!). So if you keep eating only kale and not chard or dandelion, you will end up lacking in what the chard or dandelion has that the kale doesn't... and over time that deficiency can lead to surprise illnesses. Most raw foodists hit a plateau after 5-6 years and wonder why their superpowers aren't getting any better.

My father was in the horse business. Some people have great luck raising horses while others wonder why their horses aren't doing so great. They run around in wide open pastures, eat lots of grass and yet the horses have all kinds of health problems. Why? Simple. The same as above. They have no variety. The soil under one farm is different to the soil from another. These animals are prisoners forced to eat only what is growing on that one single patch of land. The grass is only as good as what's in the soil below it. If that patch of land is lacking in selenium or cobalt or sulfur, deficiencies will arise.

In the wild, animals never stay in one place. If those horses were free and wild and there were no fences, they would be two miles away the next day munching on weeds, wild apples and grass from a whole different area with different minerals. Wild animals eat hundreds and hundreds of different things all the time. They're always moving from one place to another, which is good for many reasons. They get variety of nutrients, and because they keep moving, they never stay long enough to destroy an area (are you listening humans??). The typical person only eats maybe 15 different things from the produce section, not 300 like they are supposed to.

So, the first thing you need to do is make your trip to the food depot an adventure. Be courageous and try something different every week. You NEED to rotate! It's mandatory for successful health. Plus, if you happen to be allergic to one thing (and not know it), you won't be eating it over and over. It's safer to rotate varieties for many reasons.

LOVE YOUR ENEMY

Start by getting the things you like. I would guess that would be the sweet fruits and some token bland leafy greens. But after a little bit, you must use the rest of the stuff also, like the non-sweet fruits and bitter greens (such as kale, endive, dandelion, arugula, watercress). Go at your own pace; just know that the more bitter something is, the better it is for you. But whatever you do,

MAKE SURE YOU GET DARK LEAFY GREENS

BITTER IS BETTER

Bitter is what heals. Bitter stuff is what will save your life. The more bitter something is, the more it will enliven your liver, and your liver is where all the toxic stuff is backed up since the day your were conceived. Your liver is your filter. It's where all the bad food choices ended up, all the toxic chemicals, cigarettes, alcohol, preservatives, food additives, chlorine, flouride, heavy metals, plastic fumes, pesticides, weed killers, household cleansers, dry cleaning chemicals and fried food cholesterol ended up. Bitter plants do for a liver what a million dollar bill would do for you; they wake you up and inspire you to get to work and clean up your act. Yeah, they might not taste good, but remember it's the sugary good-tasting stuff that got you into trouble in the first place. Don't judge something by how good it tastes. Actually, usually the worse something tastes, often the better it is for you. But don't worry, I am not enslaving you to a lifetime of gastric drudgery. There are ways of making even the most nasty healing herbs palatable.

AVOID SEEDLESS

Seedless fruits and vegetables are all the rage now. Try to avoid them. They are hybrids. Man-made. High in sugars, low in nutrients and messed-up genetically. Over half the produce we buy commercially nowadays is GMO (genetically modified) by a chemical company. Don't get me started on that. All I'm going to say on that is that ultimately, my advice is to get a piece of land as far away as you can from industry and grow your own food. Encourage your neighbors to grow different things than you, so that you guys can all share year round in each others' goods. That's called a "co-op".

While you're at it, harness the power of the wind, sun, rivers and streams to power your own property for free. There are cars being developed that run on water. You can power your telephone, computer, and everything else with solar power. Oops. I got off on a tangent. Ahem.

Back to seedless. Yes. Buy only fruit with seeds. The seeds contain everything necessary for life to reproduce that plant. All the powerful nutrients, almost all the good stuff, is in the seeds and rind, not the juicy sugary part that you like. When a horse eats a melon, it eats the whole thing. Yes, it's not fun for us to bite into the rind, so that's where the Vitamix comes in. If you blend the whole watermelon - rind, seeds, everything - it actually tastes quite good!!! You'll be surprised. But MAKE SURE IT'S ORGANIC. Do not consume the rind if it's not organic, it's been sprayed with poisons. The same with other fruits; don't buy seedless grapes, seedless raisins etc.

Get lots of CELERY

Celery is one of the most underrated and most beneficial vegetables of all. It's one of the best sources of potassium, sodium and sulfur, the three most needed minerals in the human body. Also Vitamins A, B, C. It's a natural diuretic, laxative and discourages water retention, greatly improving appearance. It is a great source of natural water for hydration. Instead of drinking water (especially after the gym), drink celery juice instead. Water retention is a sign of being dehydrated, believe it or not. Make celery juice the base of every juice you make, every day.

CUCUMBER

One of the most healing fruits on Earth. Yes, it is a fruit. Really good for flushing kidneys, detoxifying the system, cleansing the bowels, digestive health, contains an enzyme that dissolves tapeworms, and has lots of calcium, magnesium, sulfur (beauty mineral) along with Vitamins E and C. Cucumber juice does wonders for complexion. Buy organic and eat the SKINS TOO, which are very high in silica, minerals and enzymes good for skin and hair.

Get a bunch of LEMONS and LIMES

Lemons are very cleansing and rich in Vitamin C and potassium. They increase digestive juices, dissolve gallstones, cleanse and rebuild the liver and are great for fasting. It is said if you drink lemon juice every day for 3 months, a clogged unhealthy liver could be cleansed and renewed. It may be wise to drink lemon juice through a straw so it doesn't melt away your tooth enamel.

PAPAYA

Papaya is one of the richest sources of natural enzymes (especially green unripe papayas), which seriously helps your digestive system, especially if you have inflamed bowels. Papayas help alleviate gas and have an enzyme that helps break down protein. Rub papaya skins on your face - the enzymes help clean away dead skin cells for a glowing complexion. Papayas have anti-tumor and anti-cancer properties. They tighten skin and help fight arteriosclerosis, strokes and heart attacks, because they contain Carpain, an alkaloid that lowers fats and cholesterol. Papayas regenerate sick, hardened livers and help get rid of parasites (especially eating the pepper-like seeds). Eat papaya every day for a week or two and feel the difference! Papaya with lemon or lime squeezed over it makes a great breakfast.

PARSLEY

Great for the lungs. It's really high in high Vitamin C and iron, so juice, blend or eat parsley whenever possible. Chewing parsley is great for bad breath. Raw parsley helps oxygen metabolism, cleanses the blood, dissolves sticky deposits in veins, maintains elasticity of blood vessels, helps move out moderately sized kidney stones and gallstones, stimulates the bowel, treats deafness and ear infections, helps sexual stuff, and stimulates the adrenals. Great for teeth, bones and helps remove heavy metals.

PUMPKIN SEEDS

A great high protein source, zinc, magnesium, B Vitamins, tryptophan. Good for treating heart disease, prostate issues, male virility and helps remove intestinal worms (roundworms, pinworms). Especially good for tapeworms. Eat a handful of raw pumpkin seeds 2 x day on an empty stomach. Even more effective (and great tasting) when mixed with garlic and a tiny bit of sea salt.

SEAWEED

Sea greens are the most nutritionally dense plants on the planet. You should have seaweed in your meals 3 x day - this stuff is a miracle food; it binds with heavy metals (like mercury) and takes them out of your body, as well as radiation. Seaweed has ten times more iron than spinach and makes hair grow like crazy, even turning gray hair dark again (if the diet is healthy). I put seaweed in my Vitamix all the time now. When there is pineapple in there too, I get a great natural sweet/salt combo taste. The main supplier of raw seaweed is Maine Coast Sea Vegetable Co. (www. SeaVeg.com). If the health store doesn't carry it, you can order online. A great source for naturally dried (not toasted or roasted) seaweeds is www. theSeaweedman.com. I get a lot of my food simply shipped to me now. Seaweed is the best source of natural iodine for healthy thyroid function. Seaweeds contain almost every mineral known to man. They are a major source of amino acids (protein). Sea greens are powerful healers. They have strong anti-inflammatory, antimicrobial, antifungal and anti-cancer properties. Sea greens are almost the only non-animal source of Vit B12. In many cases, seaweeds are more potent than the drugs used to treat breast and prostate cancer. They help heal scars and are loaded with more calcium than milk. They help get hormones and sex drive going and clear plaque out of arteries. They lower cholesterol, fight candida (yeast), cellulite, chlamydia, herpes, HIV, vaginal infections, menopause, make skin look younger and hair grow. They are rich in fiber, and packed with Vitamins, especially K, A, D, B, E, C and a broad range of carotenes. Sea vegetables should definitely be consumed every day. There is no family of foods more protective against radiation and environmental pollutants than sea vegetables.

CHIA SEEDS

Chia seeds are one of the best sources of essential fatty acids, with 2/3rds being Omega-3s (the kind we lack and need the most; these are the fats that protect against inflammation and heart disease). Chia seeds are also an excellent source of fiber, protein, vitamins, minerals, antioxidants, calcium, phosphorus, magnesium, manganese, copper, niacin and zinc.. They are very hydrating. One part chia seeds mixed with nine parts water lasts two weeks in the fridge. Chia seeds are a better source of omega-3 fatty acids than flaxseeds, and the fiber is not abrasive like flax. The Aztecs used chia to relieve joint pain and skin conditions. Chia are tiny seeds like poppy and can be eaten as is, or put in water (they turn soft on their own after a bit) or you can mix them in a blender with water or a smoothie. Chia gels into a pudding, jello consistency. It kind of tastes like a mild, instant oatmeal. A great cleanser. Great way to start and end your day, with lots of fiber and nutrition. It cleans your heart, colon and arteries while curbing your carb cravings. Chia is actually a common weed. Learn to recognize it. It's in my book "Free Food and Medicine Edible Plant Guide"

KEEP NUTS TO A MINIMUM

Don't buy flavored nuts or roasted or blanched nuts. Look for "RAW". Don't eat too many nuts, they are hard on our bodies to digest. Almond is the best choice, because it's not really a nut. It's a seed, which are better. Raw pumpkin, sesame, flax and chia seeds are great choices. All nuts and seeds (except chia, flax and cashews) need to be soaked in water for at least a few hours (preferably overnight) before using, to dissolve away the enzyme inhibitor coating which makes them difficult to digest. In the beginning it's OK to buy almond milk, almond flour etc, but down the road it's best to make your own, that way the food is much fresher and four times more nutritious. Many store-bought almond products are rancid. It only takes a minute to make anyway. Cheaper too. In the beginning you will want to make lots of sweet and salty stuff. But over time, the healthier you get, the less you will desire that, and the better you will be. For salt, the best stuff is Celtic Sea Salt. It is sea water that's been dried in the sun and then the salt is harvested by hand. It's full of sea minerals. I personally like the kind with the big chunky crystals.

Your body needs sodium, but standard table salt (pure NaCL) isn't good for you. The body needs a balanced intake of minerals. During your transition, use Celtic Sea Salt, which is harvested from the sea and has all kinds of minerals your body needs, balanced in the way they're found in nature. After a while on a raw food diet, you will get most of the sodium you need from what you eat, (like celery or seaweed) without having to add lots of salt. I add a pinch of coarse Celtic sea-salt to my food every day. Some people go completely without it.

CONDIMENTS- Beware of Sugar-White Vinegar Combo!

As for condiments, beware. The secret of most condiments is the addictive combination of sugar and vinegar. You'll find this combo in almost all sauces that you are addicted to; ketchup, mustard, relish, mayo, teriyaki, salad dressings etc. White distilled vinegar kills red blood cells and sugar is instant fuel for YEAST. Are you tired a lot? Think you have candida? Yes, breads are a yeast staple but the sugar/vinegar combo is also gasoline for the yeast fire. Remember what they use to grow virus cultures in a lab- sugar water! Nothing grows a virus or bacteria faster than sugar. Apple cider vinegar is what you should be using. To spice up your food, use real foods/spices such as raw hot peppers, cayenne, onion, fresh garlic, whatever floats your boat.

Olive Oil

Oils should be used sparingly, but a little bit here and there should be ok. The best olive oil to get is STONE CRUSHED. Even though most say "cold pressed", they are in fact pressed by a giant hydraulic mechanical press at tremendous pressure that raises the oil heat to over 160 degrees, thus ruining many of its healing properties. Look for "stone crushed" on the bottle if you can get it. It's more expensive, but worth it, otherwise why bother. You can get it at health food stores or order it from the internet. Look for brands such as Bariani. And WOW the taste! You could almost eat it like soup.

SWEETENER

For sweetener, I often just use cut up **DATES**. They are a great addiction to salads, smoothies, just about anything. They are a complete meal by themselves and very high in fiber. Mangos are a great sweetener.
Three new revolutionary sweeteners that do NOT raise the glycemic index (good for diabetics), and don't put your pancreas into shock like other sugars, are STEVIA, LO-HAN (monkfruit) and ERYTHRITOL. They

are zero calories, zero glycemic, zero insulin response, don't make you fat or feed disease and they are actually good for you. I personally think stevia tastes funky, but the other two are amazing together. I sell a healthy Lohan-Erythritol sweetener at **MarkusSweet.com** that tastes amazing.

Maple Syrup - a little is OK. Yes, it's heated, but at least it's not processed beyond that. Don't take it if you have parasites.

Agave Nectar is a sweetener made from a desert plant, and was all the rage with raw foodists when it came out, but then it was found to have almost double the fructose and is more processed than high fructose corn syrup.

On the other hand, the least amount of fructose of any sweetener is found in **pineapples** (and juice)- a much better choice.

If you have a life-threatening disease, you must stay away from sugar of any kind. This includes agave nectar, maple syrup, honey, yacon syrup, etc. We all crave flavor to our food, but we need to abstain from this for the time being while we heal, because anything you crave is also craved by parasites, cancer, viruses, bacteria, yeast, mold, fungus and anything else that grows. Eating these items gives these unwelcome visitors more energy to spread.

RAW CHOCOLATE
(for people who are not doing a serious cleanse)
Chocolate comes from a coffee-like bean called "cacao", which is the same as "cocoa". Why they renamed it into that stupid new lettering is beyond me. Anyway, you can buy the beans in their raw state, or as nibs, which is the bean without its bitter, paper-like shell, broken into bits, or as powder. In its natural state, cacao is bitter, pure 100% dark chocolate. Some chocolate die-hards eat it straight. Most take the nibs, grind them into powder at home in a coffee grinder, mix this with coconut oil, some kind of sweetener and a few other ingredients and make their own chocolate. They simply mix the ingredients by hand, put the pot in the freezer to make it hard, and an hour later break off pieces and eat it.

I have an awesome recipe on my website **FreezerChocolate.com** and in this book.

Raw chocolate is a good transition food because it has GOOD oils and fats. Commercial chocolate has bad oils and fats (hydrogenated), so that it can stay hard at room temperature and have a long shelf life. The oils in raw chocolate melt at room temp (they are liquid in your body and don't clog your arteries) and therefore need to be in the freezer to be hard until you eat it. You can also take raw chocolate powder and put it into smoothies and other dishes to make raw chocolate ice cream, dessert pies and so on. Chocolate contains a bitter alkaloid called theobromine which some people say is bad for you, but in my opinion, its not much worse for you than coffee, that bit of chocolate you're going to have isn't going to make much difference. Our uncookbook has recipes for making raw vegan versions of chocolate marzipan treats, chocolate cake, creme brulee, candy apples and amazing cookies. See? Raw food doesn't have to be boring. Some of this stuff is downright addictive. Save the chocolate and sweet stuff for AFTER the cleansing and healing though, especially if you have a life-threatening disease. It will be your reward. if you're relatively healthy, then this stuff is totally ok.

THE SUPPLEMENT SECTION

If this was the 1800s, then maybe we wouldn't have to stop by the supplement section. But all the produce we buy in grocery stores nowadays (even organic) is grown in soil that is very depleted of valuable nutrients. To get the same amount of iron as a bowl of spinach from 1950, you would have to eat FIFTY bowls of spinach nowadays. Magnesium, without which our bodies cannot absorb calcium, is so low in today's soil that it's almost not even there. Without magnesium our hearts stop working. Without magnesium, our nervous systems become frazzled, stressed-out toast. There is no more iodine in the soil. Without it, our thyroids stop working. In nature, we would eat a plant with soil organisms on it, that's where we get B12. But store produce is washed clean of all that. So, off to the supplement section we go.

Firstly, forget about multi-vitamin pills. They are useless and overburden your liver and kidneys. Three quarters of the products in the supplement section are useless. It's the same useless dead chemical isolates repackaged under different company labels, but most of it comes from the same places. I looked into it when I was formulating my own herbal products. I found that the bottling companies source their ingredients from giant warehouses, where ingredients are stored for years and years. They are dirt cheap and useless. Almost all the supplement bottles you see on the shelves cost no more than two dollars each to make - that includes the bottle, the capsules and the ingredients. On the other hand, I wanted organic or wildcrafted herbs in my formulas, and that raised the cost by as much as TEN times. That should tell you how cheap all that other stuff is. Don't be fooled by fancy labels or company names that make you think they are all-natural and healthy. Most Vitamins are made from inorganic sources like ground-up stone. Herbs are usually the cheapest available, sprayed with toxins and shipped in from some foreign country where health laws don't apply. This irritated me even more into making my own products. That's how my own line of healing products came about. I wanted to share with others what I myself was taking. Anyway, back to the supplement section at the store...

The first thing you need is **MAGNESIUM**. Almost everyone is dangerously low in magnesium nowadays, so low in fact that it can lead to heart attacks. I personally use a product called NATURAL CALM (magnesium citrate). Magnesium malate is even better. I take one teaspoon, 2 or 3 times a day with water. The reason it's called "Calm" is because magnesium makes you feel calm. It's great for soothing stress and nerves. It's great for heart, kidneys and restful sleep. It calms hyperactive children, helps diabetes, blood pressure, arthritis, migraines, asthma, hormones, hair loss and greying, depression, joint problems, pain, leg cramps, muscle spasms, increases sexual energy and is a major preventer of strokes. Next to oxygen, magnesium is the most important substance in the body. We need lots of it. Without magnesium, calcium cannot be absorbed into the body. If other healing methods aren't working that should be working, it means you are low in magnesium.

69

e needed for every bodily function. They are the spark of life. ̃ss you have, the shorter your life. Your body cannot use vitamins without minerals, and cannot use minerals without protein (amino acids), and cannot use protein without enzymes. Take them when you eat bad food, heavy amounts of protein, or feel run down, but don't go crazy with them or your body will stop making it's own.

CHIA and FLAX SEEDS for your Omega-3 EFAs . Chia tastes kinda like instant jello oatmeal when mixed in a blender with water. A few spoonfuls of flax seeds a day will give you enough Omega 3. Grind them into a powder in a coffee grinder and add to smoothies or salads.

Yes, it's true we need MultiVitamins to make up for what we are lacking, but don't go for the pill form. Go for mother nature.

Look for **CHLORELLA** as your Multi-vitamin. (a better choice than Spirulina) Algaes are considered some of the most complete foods on the planet - you can live off the stuff indefinitely. It has ALL the amino acids (complete protein), more than any other whole food on Earth (62% protein), plus all kinds of minerals, enzymes, chlorophyll and pretty much everything else... Beta carotene (Vit A), C, E, K, B complex B1, B2, B6, B12, niacin, pantothenic acid, RNA, DNA, folic acid, biotin, choline, and inositol. Phosphorus, potassium, magnesium, germanium, sulfur, iron, calcium, manganese, copper, zinc, iodine, cobalt, and trace elements. It replicates so fast that it quadruples every twenty-four hours (amazing genetics). It also quadruples our friendly flora (probiotics), making it one of the most potent 'growth factors' available (listen up bodybuilders). It boosts the immune system immensely (helps children grow and stay healthy), helps digestion, alkalizes, heals intestinal lining, helps remove chemicals, toxins and heavy metals from the body. It enhances health and muscle growth, increases the concentration of hemoglobin in red blood cells (for iron and oxygen), helps reduce cholesterol, and helps the liver detox. I know I mentioned chlorella before, but it's worth repeating. Best taken on an empty stomach at least twenty minutes before other food. You can also just get my green formula which has Chlorella and several dozen other of the most powerful plant sources for super nutrition.

Also while you're in the cold section of the supplement area, be sure to grab a jar of **liquid PROBIOTICS**. These are living bacteria that live in your intestines and do everything from helping break down food to fighting bacteria and disease, while keeping the place clean. These are super important for health. When our bodies become run down from eating bad food or even just being stressed, the beneficial bacteria (called "flora") get killed and we lose our barrier of protection down there. You will need probiotics also when you do colonics or enemas, to replenish the ones you wash out. Take early morning or before bed with water. The best kind of probiotics are the live cultures kept alive in things like coconut milk and fruit juice or fermented foods. Get the liquid kind of probiotics, not the capsules. They are often useless. Order some **KEFIR GRAIN**S online and grow your own cultures. You'll never run out! PREBIOTICS is the term for what probiotics eat... and the best probiotic food is FIBER. A good one is FOS (Fructooligosaccharides)

Get a bottle of raw, unfiltered **APPLE CIDER VINEGAR**. This is good for cleaning your body from the inside, and also building stomach acid. Take two tablespoons every morning in water. Add to salads as dressing with some oil.

Get some **GREEN TEA or WHITE TEA**. White tea is like green tea, but more powerful. This will be your new coffee. It dilates your blood vessels, makes you feel really good and helps fight disease, even cancer.

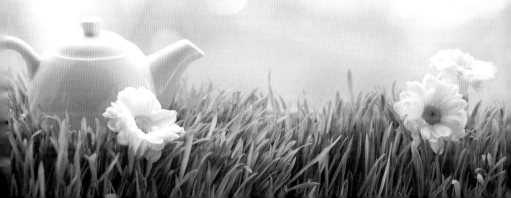

TOCOTRIENOLS (rice bran solubles)

You will feel the difference... This is a light, fluffy, great-tasting powder made from rice that you mix with water. It's a good source of complete B vitamins, vitamin E, all necessary amino acids, minerals, essential fatty acids, and over 70 antioxidant compounds. It's hypoallergenic, easy on the digestive system and adds significant fiber to the diet. It reduces cholesterol, regulates diabetic blood glucose, suppresses cancer tumor cells, enhances immune system responsiveness, is great for youthful skin, reduces renal calcium excretion related to kidney stones and increases bile acid binding in the gallbladder. This is a great "protein powder" that you can take as a whole meal replacement if you are crunched for time or while traveling; great to have while on the road.

PERSONAL CARE

While at the health food store, get some all-natural cleaning stuff, such as dishwashing liquid and veggie-wash spray made with citrus. Also, get the most natural laundry detergent you can find. Bleach can be replaced with safer sodium percarbonate or hydrogen peroxide. The acid water produced by alkaline water machines is awesome for cleaning and disinfecting dishes, countertops and laundry. (The ACID water, not the alkaline water!) As for hair products, make sure they have no Sodium Lauryl Sulfate or anything like that. You can use apple cider vinegar as your shampoo and conditioner. Try it! You'll be amazed. For teeth and gums, you can make your own tooth powder with baking soda, sea salt and cayenne. Wash mouth with hydrogen peroxide. No more bleeding gums! (That bacteria in your mouth that cause bleeding, by the way, are a leading cause of heart disease and dramatically shortening people's lives.) Make sure you get your teeth cleaned regularly-without flouride.

Not everything you get at a health food store is organic. Sometimes we have no choice but to buy non-organic, in which case, go get these items somewhere else cheaper. One great place to get stuff really inexpensively is Asian markets. Almost every town has one. That's where I get my white **YOUNG THAI COCONUTS**. They are almost three dollars each at the health food store, but at the Asian market right around the corner, I can buy a box of NINE for FIVE dollars!!! And guess what? They are the very same. There is presently no such thing as organic or non-organic Thai coconuts, they are all imported from the same place. Asian markets are also the best place to buy GINGER, because they have so much of it available. I fill a whole bag with it.

Asian markets are also where to buy **DURIAN**, a weird alien-looking fruit the size of a turkey with sharp spiky thorns all over it. It smells really funky but the taste is amazing. Inside, it has a custard-like filling that tastes just like custard pudding and when mixed in a blender with some coconut juice and meat, wow: instant dessert heaven. But the cool thing about raw food is that the dessert can be your main course! You can see me demonstrating it at DurianRecipe.com. Durians are very high in protein (good for muscle building) and VERY GOOD FOR YOU. They are high in tryptophan (good for depression, insomnia) and sulfur (hence the smell) They are very, very addictive. I get the frozen kind because they don't smell as strongly as the unfrozen ones. I let the durian thaw overnight and prepare it in the morning.

Asian markets are a great place to find exotic, interesting fruit and vegetables not found anywhere else. Try it all! Life is an adventure, not a chore.

Tip: don't get lots of starchy roots. Try to keep most of your diet to what grows ABOVE THE GROUND. Starchy roots are hard to digest and full of concentrated sugars. You want the green stuff that grows on top, not the starchy stuff underneath. Plant starches are better than animal products, but if you look at many heavy cooked-starch eaters, they seem to age faster and get sick more than raw vegans. So at least while cleansing and healing, stay with things that grow above the ground, like the greens.

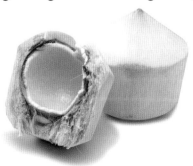

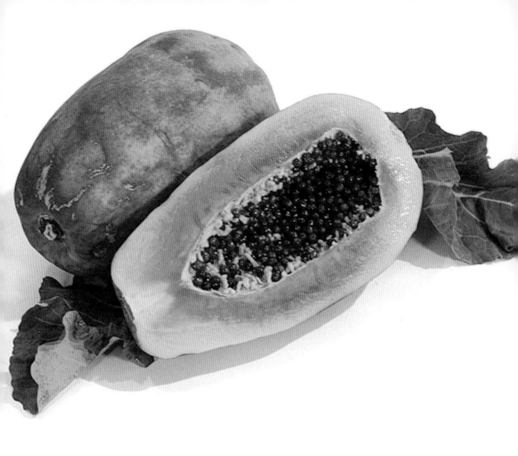

PAPAYA

Papayas are very rich in enzymes (especially green ones) making them great for digestion and glowing skin.The enzymes immediately set to work tightening our skins collagen tissue. Papaya has anti-tumor and anti-cancer properties- it's enzymes eat cancer proteins. Papayas also reduce the risk of arteriosclerosis, strokes, and heart attacks because it contains Carpain, an alkaloid which lowers the concentration of fats and cholesterol in the blood stream. It also helps regenerate a hardened, dysfunctional liver. Papaya seeds help get rid of parasites- eat 1 tablespoon seeds each day for a week (chew well), then wait a week, then eat again for another week. Papaya seeds can be added to salad dressing for black-pepper-like spice. This amazing fruit is used to improve digestion, alleviate gas, prevent and heal ulcers, treat cancer and reduce inflammation.

OK, let's take our groceries home and I'll show you what to do with them. (No, we aren't going to stop by Starbucks to get a cappuccino and muffin on the way)... but we ARE going to stop by the corner drug store and buy an ENEMA bag. Not those little stupid disposable plastic things. You want the one that's a rubber bag that holds half a gallon of water with a tube running out of it. At the end of the tube are tips that you can switch out. This is a multi-purpose item used for douching, enemas or simply as a hot water bottle. While you're here, get several gallons of SPRING WATER. If you can't find an enema bag, order one online.

BOWLS and POTS: **USE ONLY GLASSWARE** (like Pyrex).

Definitely don't use any non-stick anything. It's deadly toxic. If you had a bird nearby while heating a non-stick pan, the fumes would kill the bird. Definitely don't use aluminum, it's one of the main causes of Alzheimer's. Try not to use metal items. Stainless steel contains nickel, a poisonous metal. We have enough heavy metals in our system as it is, another reason to not use metal forks and spoons. They react negatively with our body, both electrically and chemically. Many people get heavy metal poisoning from their knives and forks while they try to eat healthily and detox. Every time they slide that spoon or fork in and out of their mouth, they are absorbing all kinds of metals such as nickel which is used in stainless steel and is very toxic. There are some new types of utensils coming out, from bamboo to disposable, Earth-friendly potato-cornstarch based items.

DISINFECTANTS (for washing fruit, veggies, hands, mouth, gums etc): **Hydrogen Peroxide**. Or add a few drops of Thyme Oil to water. Just don't get it in your eyes - that stuff is powerful! Thyme is used in developing countries to disinfect questionable drinking water. Acids disinfect, like vinegar or acid water from pH machines.

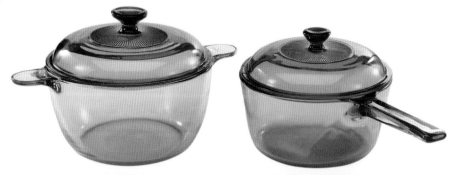

And lastly, 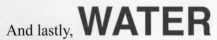 **WATER**

You are three-quarters water. Well, actually you are mainly just energy and air, but we'll discuss that later. For now, I'm talking in old-school thinking that people can understand.

Water. Water. Water. You are a gooey blob of stuff and without water you would be a small dry pile of minerals on the ground. Water is more than just H2o (hydrogen and oxygen). Firstly, the body is a big battery filled with around 18 gallons of salt water solution that gives us life. Water conducts electricity. Water is a universal supercomputer. What science is finding out about water is enough to make our mouths drop and to rip wide open everything we understand about God and the Universe. Water has memory. Water communicates. Water has energy. It is literally a universal liquid supercomputer. Many scientific studies have been done all over the world on water, such as these I am about to tell you about...

If you have two glasses of water, and you send loving thoughts into one and hateful angry thoughts into the other... and then you give that second glass to someone to drink, they would probably become ill, whereas the first glass would make them feel good without them knowing why. Water carries emotions, thoughts, energy and data across time and space. You and I are water. Water connects all things on this planet. Your breath has water vapor that I inhale. The air we breathe has water in it. The water we drink came from someone else's body at some time... actually from billions of people, with all their thoughts, emotions and energies. There is so much significance to us being well and harmonious, because we are all literally one. Science is proving this. Read the book "The Genie in Your Genes", by Dawson Church, Ph.D. This is radical stuff. We are on the very edge of a new way of living and being. Epigenetics is now proving that our DNA is actually changed by our thoughts. We literally create ourselves and our future.

Anyway, back to water (there is so much to talk about, it's hard to control myself sometimes). Ahem. Water. Bottom line: we need to make sure the water we drink is clean and not messed up energetically or else we become messed up. There are so many things that mess up water... bacteria and parasites, or poisons, heavy metals and plastics. Then there's the ionic charge. Like everything else, water is made of atoms and molecules that have an electrical charge. If there aren't enough electrons, water sucks them from us. Water also needs a proper molecular structure.

In the glorious days of past when nature was clean, the water that came out of springs was virgin perfect healing water. Nowadays, we drink out of plastic bottles and from rusty old pipes filled with slime, mold, bacteria, poisons and rusty metal. Even if we filter it, it is dead, unstructured water, lacking proper electron charge. Stay away from alkaline water- it neutralizes your stomach acid creating all kinds of problems, like runaway yeast, fungus, H.Pylori, undigested food, etc. Actually, do the opposite- a little lemon or apple cider vinegar for acid.

Water in plastic bottles is a big huge no-no. Plastic is an estrogenic that leads to breast cancer and all kinds of problems. It also makes the water taste bad. Try to fill up your water from a good source in reusable glass bottles. There is a website called FindASpring.com that helps you find a natural spring in your area. I get mine delivered in 5 gallon bottles from a company called Mountain Valley Spring Water. If you are on a low budget, there are water machines outside most grocery stores where you can fill up your own bottles for 75 cents per gallon (real cheap). They use a five-stage filtration system including ultraviolet, carbon and Reverse Osmosis. Take gallon sized glass bottles (not plastic) if you can. The best way to get gallon sized glass bottles is re-using big gallon-sized apple juice bottles. Throw out the dead pasteurized apple juice and now you have an awesome reusable glass water jug! The best water is spring water. Go find a spring if you can because spring water is best.

I also suggest getting a whole-house water filtration system to filter out chlorine, chemicals, toxins and bacteria. Chlorine knocks out the thyroid.

brand shown: Excalibur

DEHYDRATOR

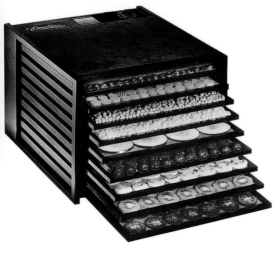

This is the first thing many people get when they go raw because it helps them make firm or dry crunchy foods like cookies, raw "breads", coconut macaroons, kale chips, raw burgers and all kinds of other texture-appeasing goodies. Dehydrators heat food, but not over 118 degrees F (45 Celsius), so the enzymes don't get killed. Dehydration takes all the moisture out of the food, making patties that can be taken on the road, to work, or munched on while around the house or watching TV. But, because they are dehydrated, these items try to re-hydrate inside your body, meaning they need moisture from your body, so drink lots of water. It's ok to eat dehydrated food occasionally, just control yourself. Remember dehydrated food is dry. Everything in your body has to be turned into liquid (blood), so it take more energy to digest and absorb dehydrated food than fresh fruit. Nothing is better than wet juicy plant food plucked right from nature. Dehydrated food in my opinion should be a backup to be used occasionally when needed or desired, but not on a regular basis. Stick to the fresh, water-rich foods in their natural state as much as possible. Remember, we are wet moist gooey beings, so eat food that's wet moist and gooey.

OK, that should about cover the basics. Your kitchen should be stocked now and ready for action. But before you start putting all that good stuff in your body, you need to make room for it, or else it won't do you much good.

You need to clean out your body first. Grab that filtered spring water and it's off to the bathroom we go...

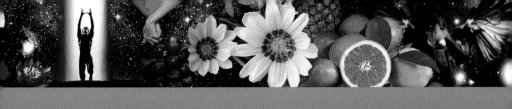

CLEANING OUT

THE MOST IMPORTANT STEP OF ALL

Without this, all the great healthy nutrition in the world does you no good.

It's like putting great gasoline in a rusted out, gunked-up car. You NEED to clean out your pipes! No excuses, no delay. This is your FIRST STEP and you CAN'T bypass it if you want serious results.

The cheap cheater way is to simply take a couple tablespoons Epsom Salts with warm water to get things moving, or take a colon cleansing formula. They work OK, but not anywhere near as well as some good ol' serious colon/bowel irrigation with lots of water.

Water is the universal cleanser and you need to wash yourself clean INSIDE as well as outside. It's kind of ironic how many "neat freaks" that keep their house spotless are actually filthy and rotting away on the inside.

ENEMA
THE MIRACLE CLEANER

If there was just one thing out of all of this that I would say was the most important over anything else, I would say it is this: an enema bag. It's also the cheapest healing device anywhere. For under ten dollars, you can 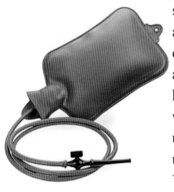 save your life. If you have food poisoning, a splitting sinus headache, constipation, diarrhea, feel tired and sluggish, feel depressed and run down, feel a cold coming on, or have ANYTHING wrong with you, this will amaze you. Sure, it makes you squeam uncomfortably at the thought of putting water up your butt, but hey, IT'S ONLY WATER! You wash your car, you wash your laundry, you roto-rootered your house, you cleaned out the fuel injectors and fuel lines in your car... isn't it about time you washed YOURSELF??? When was the last time you washed out your own plumbing? Never? And you wonder why you are so sluggish and run down?

By the way, the type of enema I am referring to is like the one in this picture, not the small disposable kind that has toxic chemicals in it. This is where your healing starts. Right here in your bathroom.

Here's what you need...

-rubber enema bag (hot water bottle type)
-hose with plastic enema tip
-at least a half gallon of body temperature warm clean filtered water (spring water or flat mineral water is better than distilled because distilled could cause an electrolyte imbalance)
-bit of coconut or olive oil to lubricate tip
-a toilet
-thirty minutes

*note: if you have money, you might want to do a series of COLONICS, which means you go to a professional place to have colon cleansing done for you. It's more comfortable, but costs probably 60 dollars or so per visit. At least an enema you can do in the privacy of your own bathroom, for mere pennies. The colonic keeps pushing water in and out of you for an entire hour, so in theory, a colonic is more thorough than an enema, but if you do it the way I advise, you can get pretty darn good results on your own at home, especially if you keep doing it regularly. I personally prefer enemas over colonics.

How To Do an Enema
This could save a life.

All you need is an enema bag (see image above), at least half a gallon of filtered luke-warm water and some kind of lubricant (preferably natural, like coconut oil or olive oil).

If the bag is brand new, wash it out a few times to get rid of the fumes. Warm the water to body temperature, fill the rubber enema bag and attach the hose. Let a bit of water run out to get rid of air bubbles. Pinch the hose and lubricate the tip. Hang the bag upside down (they come with a hook), on something that will be higher than you. A good suggestion is to hang it on a towel rack near the toilet, kneel down on the floor, insert the tip in your butt, and then put your face on the ground with your butt in the air- to work properly, your rear end needs to be HIGHER THAN YOUR STOMACH, and the water bottle needs to be higher than your butt (see diagram). See the video about how to do an enema at Enema101.com

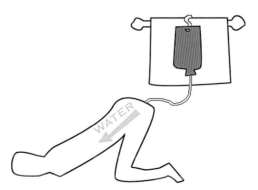

You might have to wiggle around to get things started. Have your hand on the hose so that you can pinch it to stop the water flow if needed. If this is your first time ever, you'll probably have some freaky, paranoid "oh my God" moments, like the first time you had sex... you'll probably think "is it supposed to feel like this?", "am I going to burst?", etc... don't worry, it's only water and you will not burst. Look at all the grossly overweight people out there; if their guts can get to be four feet across then surely you can handle a little water. When the water starts going in you will first feel an overwhelming urge to go to the bathroom; resist this urge as much as you can. Pinch the hose and relax for a moment. Breathe. But if you absolutely have to let it out, then pinch the hose, pull out the tip and hop on the toilet to let it out. Then continue. Each time, you should get a little more water in. Keep going. Refill the bag again. Keep doing this until you can get in a WHOLE BAG (half a gallon of water, 3.8L), all at once. The cleaner you are, the easier this gets. It will get to the point where the water runs in fast and you don't even feel it.

If you feel the urge to go to the bathroom immediately after starting this, with only a tiny bit of water in you, that means you are not clean and healthy. You are either clogged up with a blockage of crap-ola, or you have IBS (irritable bowel syndrome). Whatever the reason or cause, get as much water in there as you can, then let it out into the toilet, then put MORE water in... etc, etc. Each time you should get more water in, meaning you are getting in deeper and cleaning things up. You have a lot of crap to dissolve. Keep going, refilling the bag until you can get a whole bag in at once. Each time it should get easier and easier. That's a sign things are better and your body is cleaner.

Maybe nothing is happening and no water is flowing; probably blocked. wiggle your body and the hose and the tip to help the water find its way through your plumbing and keep going until the bag is empty. Again, don't let the urge to go to the bathroom stop you, keep going if you can. After a few times you will get used to it and master it. Some people distract themselves by singing or yelling stupid jokes or simply making loud baby sounds, whatever works. Empty that bottle!

Another good way to help things along is to blow all the air out of your lungs, as if you were blowing up a balloon. This raises your diaphragm and causes a vacuum inside your intestines, helping suck the water in. Take another breath and blow out again with a big long slow HOOOOOOOMPH, and help suck the water in. Or you can just sing. Personally I like to do Richard Nixon impersonations. Hey, with the side of your head pressed against the bathroom floor with your butt high in the air, you end up saying some silly things :-). Once the water starts going - it shouldn't take more than a minute or two - look at the bag to see if it's fully deflated and flat.

When you are done, pull out the tip and go to the toilet. If you think you can hold it, lie down on your side and roll around. Rub your belly. Jump up and down. The idea is to swish the water around to loosen years of hardened crap, just like a pot in your kitchen sink that has black burnt food stuck to it - you need to soak it in water to loosen it. I hang on an inversion table upside down so that the water runs all the way up through the colon. This is what "high colonic" means. I swing up and down, back and forth so it sloshes all through me and loosens crap. Then I jump up and down and rub my abs. When you can't hold it any more, go to the toilet and let it all out. Stay there because you should have about five more waves in the next twenty minutes, each time being a major bowel movement. That's right, five big dumps in half an hour, WOW you will be amazed! I never get results like that with even a pro colon hydrotherapist.

This is where the magic happens. As the old garbage comes out below, many people instantly feel their heads clear up (headaches, sinus congestion etc), and fresh air fills the inside of their head. Sometimes it takes several sessions to get to that, but just like that crusty pot in your kitchen sink, the longer you soak and the more times you do it, the more old crap you get rid of. Remember, you're not going to get rid of 40 years of crust in one day, but water is the universal solvent. It is the easiest, cheapest and by far the safest way to CLEAN OUT!!!

I have an enema available at MarkusEnema.com

I suggest a couple of times in a row for people not feeling well. if you're really sick, I suggest at least one enema per day. Once you are well, twice a month for regular maintenance is what I do.

After a good cleansing, take probiotics - these are friendly organisms naturally found in your intestines that help break down food and fight disease. If you get lots of cleansing sessions, these probiotics help replace the good stuff that gets washed out. Don't worry too much about being "depleted" of good stuff if you are consuming fresh RAW fruits, vegetables and juices like you are supposed to, because these foods already contain all the good stuff.

WHAT IS A COLONIC ?

A colonic is where you pay someone to do colon hydrotherapy for you (although some of the newer places have colonic systems where you can do the treatment yourself). It's like a luxury treatment enema. You lay on a table with a gown, a hose is discretely inserted and a technician has a machine that regulates the flow of water (which is at body temperature, so you barely feel anything). The water goes in and then you simply let go... it goes out through an exit hose and new water is let in and so on. This in-out cycle goes for about an hour. It's more thorough than an enema and more relaxing. The lights are usually dimmed and they play soft music like being at a spa getting a massage. These people are professionals and see rear-ends all day long - most of them probably uglier than yours, so don't worry. They chose that job and be thankful they did because these people have truly chosen to help others - these people are, in my opinion, unselfish healers who do ten times more good than money-hungry doctors who dispense pills to hide symptoms. Washing yourself out with water doesn't just hide symptoms, it helps get RID of your old illness-causing stuff. No matter what you have that's bad in you - poisons, bad food, bacteria, viruses, gallstones, cholesterol, alien implants - it all gets sent to your internal garbage can and if the colon is not clean, then this crap gets stuck in the crevices and stays there for years, making you sick, sluggish and not able to function properly. If you have the money, pay these people what you would pay a doctor. Seriously. They do more good than doctors.

I suggest also taking Chanca Piedra, a South American herb whose name literally translates to "Stone Breaker", which dissolves gall and kidney stones. It's in my liver formula.   Now all you have to do is help wash them out... with... you guessed it- enemas or colonics.

QUICK FIXES

I always take an enema bag with me when I travel on any trip over three days long, because I know IT WORKS. I'm ready for anything.
But if you are squeamish and don't like the thought of enemas, in a pinch you can always take with you some of my Colon Formula (available at MarkusProducts.com). Or simply go to any grocery or drug store and get some Epsom Salts and put a couple tablespoons in a glass of warm water and you will be high-tailing it to the toilet in no time. It tastes really really really bad though. Epsom Salts is nothing more than a form of magnesium (sulfate) and your body welcomes magnesium.The next step depends on how sick you are. If you have no apparent health issues and just want to get sexier, then just do a bunch of enemas while starting your raw food regimen.

But for the REST of you, my suggestion is that no matter who you are and how healthy you think you are, ALL OF YOU should do what is discussed in the following section, because if you want a serious life change, this is how you do it. Even if you are healthy, this will take you to new heights of amazing health, sexual vitality and spiritual awareness that you never knew possible. Whatever level of health you are at, the following will take you higher.

MUCH higher!

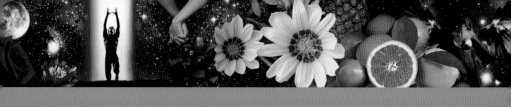

FASTING

THE UNIVERSAL HEALER

I"F FASTING CAN'T HEAL IT, IT PROBABLY CAN'T BE HEALED."
Somebody Famous

Every major healer and religion throughout history says to do this. So obviously there is something to it. And trust me... there is!

Most people have no idea how important this is and that fasting is one of the best things you can do for yourself. It has been said that fasting alone can heal almost anything. What is fasting? It means to not eat or drink anything except water or lemon juice or green juice. What does it do? It gives your digestive system a chance to rest and since most of your body's energy goes into digesting food, this gives your body a chance to take all that energy and put it towards housecleaning instead. When we don't eat, our body starts putting attention on cleaning out the poisons and waste stored in our tissues and cells. During a fast, disease, tumors, lumps and even parasites starve and die because they have no more food source. We personally have nothing to worry about because our cells contain enough nutrition to last a long time, especially if we keep taking in water (with maybe a bit of lemon juice) or fresh vegetable juice. Angela Stokes is famous for her 92 day juice "feast", healing people with consuming nothing but vegetable juice for 3 months. But we don't need to be that radical. Depending on how sick you are, I am suggesting one week to a month on juice before moving on to blended drinks.

As a general rule, never eat anything anyway if you are not hungry or if you are sick or in pain. Just drink water and fresh vegetable juices. It is the best and most natural way to get and stay healthy.

To someone on the outside who's never done this, the first thoughts are "oh my god, I'll get skinny and can't eat my favorite foods, I'll waste away, I'll have no energy, I won't be able to work, I'll get weak and possibly sick, bla bla bla". Right? That's your sick paranoid food-addicted mind. It's scared and trying to give you a million reasons not to do this. First of all, none of that is true. Secondly, the reason your chattery mind is saying all that is because it will cease to exist on the cleanse. While fasting, one becomes amazingly peaceful and all worries go away. Our minds stop chattering. We become at peace with ourselves, as a beautiful serene sense of being bathes our soul like morning sunlight warms darkness.

Yes, you will lose weight, but what you lose is nothing healthy, only fat, toxic crap and anything your body doesn't need or want. Your body isn't stupid. If you've been living off pizza, coffee, pasta, meat, potatoes, bread, cheese, fast food and carbonated soda, then yes, you will lose a lot of weight and size, because most of you is GARBAGE - that's what your cells are made of. All of that will be stripped away first before rebuilding. It's just like how a car or house is rebuilt: strip it down to the frame and then rebuild properly. That's what fasting is all about. You strip down to the frame, before rebuilding. Men are afraid they will lose their precious manly muscles. Yet that one step back will help you leap two steps forward: you will be amazed how fast you get your size back, and this time it will be REAL muscle, not fluffy water muscle like before. You won't get sore after workouts and your strength will double.

Getting thin is a little sacrifice to make for a month or two considering that you have a lifetime of great looks and super health ahead of you. If you don't lose weight while fasting or going raw...

...that means your body is toxic. When people go raw, the body dumps all kinds of toxins that have been accumulating in the cells over your lifetime. This is a major housecleaning, and sometimes the body has more toxins and acids than it can flush out naturally, so new fat cells are created as a protective storage mechanism to store the toxins. Fat is a defensive measure. If you are eating all raw foods and still having trouble losing weight, then you are toxic and not removing the toxins, meaning you are not doing your bowel cleansing enough (enemas, colonics etc), and not exercising enough either. Eat only raw fresh juicy foods, juice lots of greens, reduce stress, drink lots of healthy water and move your body to burn the calories. It could also mean the thyroid and adrenals are burned out from stress and lack of iodine (seaweed is a good source of natural iodine). Be asleep by 9 or 10 pm.

As for energy, during a fast, you actually HAVE TONS MORE ENERGY! You will be amazed. Most people are astounded how after six hours sleep they can't stay in bed anymore. They are up at the first rays of light, bouncing off the walls with energy they never felt since they were kids... and they think "how is this possible? I'm not eating. Where is all this energy coming from???" And thus begins the new awakening. A new understanding starts to dawn upon the newly initiated that massive energy and health has nothing to do with how much food you stuff into your face. Actually, it's quite the opposite. How much food do you think a hummingbird eats? As a matter of fact, do you think they even eat at all? Their mouth is a tiny thin needle, used to suck liquid from plants. What are you doing during a juice fast? Sucking in liquid from plants!

Fasting is the best medicine of all. Try it for at least three days, shoot for a week. Many serious people live off nothing but water, lemon and green juices for months and months and heal almost anything you can think of.

Fasting is the best way to get toxins, poisons, disease and waste out of your body and it gives the body a chance to heal internal wounds. Without a fast, the body never has a chance to do deep cleansing. During a fast, disease, parasites, tumors, lumps, and bad stuff has to compete for nutrients with our organs, and our body makes sure that our organs win. Studies show that no protein is lost during a 24 hour fast, only fat and bad stuff. Fasting helps get rid of weak old stuff and boosts the production of new cells. For serious anti-aging and health results do a 24 hour fast one day a week every week, for the rest of your life. One recommendation is to start fasting after lunch and go until lunch the next day.

For people who are overweight or want to heal a health condition or simply become reborn, I seriously suggest a fast.

All you are consuming the entire time of the fast is juice, water, tea and some herbs. That's it. The juice will have all the minerals, Vitamins and enzymes you need.

My personal recommendation is to do a two-day water fast and then do a juice fast for a week to a month, depending on what you are trying to heal, then switch to another few weeks of nothing but BLENDED drinks (which includes the fiber), then slowly reintroduce solid raw fruits and vegetables while continuing the blended drinks.

Stop consuming any juice at least two or three hours before bed. Only water. Make sure you get lots of sleep while fasting - be in bed by 10 pm for best effectiveness. 9 is better. Healing hormones are released between 10 pm and 2 am and you need to be asleep for this to work.

During the the fast, do bowel cleansing, because the entire time of the fast your body is dumping all the toxins you have been accumulating during your lifetime into your bloodstream, lymph system and elimination organs and you need to help the body get rid of that heavy load, otherwise you are re-poisoning yourself.

At first during a fast, you may experience detox symptoms like tiredness, headaches, lightheadedness, weakness, nausea, vomiting, stomach cramps, body odor, bad breath, back and kidney pain. The more you've abused your body over the years, the more detox symptoms you will have. Remember this is garbage coming out of you and making you feel funky, not a side effect of fasting. Celebrate that the bad stuff is coming out, never to weight you down again. Even bad thoughts, fears, insecurities, repressed resentment and anger come to the surface before leaving you. You end up SO MUCH LIGHTER, you will be amazed how light a human being can feel. You'll feel like part of the air.

All you'll hear is the song of the universe playing in your heart.

Fasting does not just clean out your cells. It cleans out the ENERGY in your cells, meaning any negative energy... yes that's right, I'm talking about emotions. Fasting gives the cells, the nervous system, the brain... everything, a physiological rest. Dr. Yuri Nikolayev has been treating people with neuropsychiatric disorders in Moscow for half a century with fasting and a healthy diet. So if you are ever depressed, sick, sluggish, confused, emotionally messed up, overwhelmed, nauseous... FAST!!!! Let the body concentrate on cleaning house.

Your brain will clear up, you will think clearer and be more calm and focused.

This is a beautiful personal awakening. Many people are kind of stunned and speechless at this new feeling because they are not familiar with it. That's why during a fast, it's best to withdraw into your own quiet personal world... don't plan on going out and partying or hanging out with noisy active people and please don't watch any TV. This is a time of deep reflection, awakening and renewal. If people don't understand what you are doing or can't honor or respect your space, avoid them during this time. This is a deeply sacred time. Honor it. You are a new child being born.

Fasting not only gives your body a rest and cleaning, it also gives your brain and nervous system a rest and cleaning. Many physiological problems have been cleared up by simply fasting. Schizophrenia for example is often caused by a biochemical imbalance and that can be corrected by fasting - the body (and brain) does serious house-cleaning and puts everything back into place like it's supposed to be. Fasting has an amazing success rate at eliminating anxiety, neuroses and depression when nothing else helped. Mental clarity becomes crystal clear. A beautiful sense of peace washes over our being. We become centered again.

If you are on medication and doctor-prescribed drugs, you should consult with your doctor first because many medications require food. Everything is stronger on an empty stomach. Try to get off the meds! I hope your doctor has at least a tiny bit of empathy for you and understands your desire to get healthy. The catch is that most doctors don't want their patients to take matters into their own hands, because what if something goes wrong and they sue the doctor? Or even worse, what if the person gets well and the doctor loses a patient? There goes his vacation to Mexico. The only one who should be monitoring how you feel and deciding your life's actions is YOU. I am merely telling you what has helped millions of people throughout history. Your doctor is giving you drugs that have only been around for twenty years and have terrible side effects. Drugs don't cure anything. They only cause more problems. Get off the drugs now. Another reason for supervision is if you are on prescription medication, unfortunately, some of them require food in your stomach. You can't really heal completely if you are on medication or drugs, so your first priority is to get off them. You might experience withdrawal pains, but know that once you clean out your body, your health conditions will improve. You have to give it a chance!

FASTING AND GETTING OFF DRUGS AND MEDICATION

If you are on recreational drugs or prescription medicine, then try to stop as fast as you safely can, but if you are on seriously heavy medications that require gradual tapering down to get off them, its best not to fast during this period because the detox would be too strong, so eat food while you gradually reduce the drugs and medications - the food helps slow down the detox effects. Then when you are off the drugs/meds, you can do a serious fast/cleanse to get the toxins out of your cells, and there will be a lot because your cells and tissues are like little sponges soaked in all that stuff.

MAINTENANCE FASTING

For serious anti-aging and health results, do a 24 hour fast one day a week for the rest of your life. One recommendation is to start after lunch and go until lunch the next day. During a 24 hour fast, you lose mainly only fat and bad stuff. Energy, mental clarity and mood are dramatically improved the next day. Twice a year you should do a week-long fast during season changes (spring and fall), for the same reasons you do spring cleaning in your house. While fasting, it's good to clean out the parasites while you're at it. They are a hidden cause of half the health problems people have.

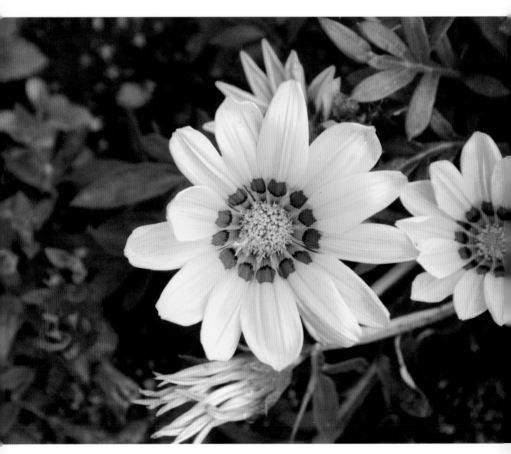

PARASITES

EVERYBODY HAS THEM

Yes, you have parasites. It's practically impossible to not come in contact with them. As a matter of fact, you couldn't live without billions of organisms inside you. The tricky part is making sure that the good outnumber the bad and the bad ones don't multiply. Everyone needs to do a parasite cleanse once or twice a year. Parasites are everywhere: doorknobs, keyboards, restrooms, shopping carts, shaking people's hands, fingernails, water, air, food, pets, walking barefoot, etc. Once they are in you, they multiply like crazy. Roundworms can lay 300,000 eggs in one day! Tapeworms can grow to be 30 feet long. Single-celled amoebas can start digesting your brain. No one is totally immune, not even the healthiest people alive. Everyone should do a parasite cleanse at least once a year. Parasites sometimes eat more of your food than you! Then they poop it into your bloodstream, lungs, organs, making you sick. Parasites can be the actual cause of most mysterious illnesses. Tired a lot? Not feeling quite right? Craving foods you KNOW are bad for you? Irritable? Cramps? Bloating? Gas? Hungry all the time? Sore, stiff joints? Breathing problems? Itching? Memory cloudy? Guess who's causing it!

Parasites can be the culprit behind almost every medical condition known. Our bodies are veritable breeding grounds for bacteria, yeast, mold, fungus, viruses and parasites. You may think you're clean on the outside. But wait till you see what's inside you! See some really nasty pictures at NastyParasites.com

Yes, cooking and boiling food kills most parasites. The irony is cooked food doesn't contain parasites but it FEEDS them. What you consume has a lot to do with keeping parasites alive. They want to live. The gross images you see on NastyParasites.com, where they are pulling spaghetti-like worms out of people's stomachs, are taken in China where people eat cooked vegetables and rice.

Parasites slowly eat away at your organs and poop toxic waste into your system! Everybody has them. They are on doorknobs, shopping carts, public places, PETS... even shaking someone's hand can transfer half a million organisms (they breed under the fingernails). Most medical problems are parasite-related. Worms can release up to A MILLION eggs per day depending on their type! They eat your food and they eat YOU. Do not be in denial of this before it's too late.

Roundworms alone for example can lay 300,000 eggs in ONE DAY! Do you eat sushi? One square inch of raw meat such as sushi can contain up to 10,000 parasite eggs and larvae! Not all parasites are big worms, many are so tiny that you can't see them. These things are EVERYWHERE inside us: in our blood, just under our skin, in our organs, and totally clogging our digestive system, making it difficult for food and fecal matter to pass through.

Oh the fun gets better. Did you know that more than half of your poop is not your own? That's right - it's poop from bacteria, worms and organisms living inside you! They eat and poop just like us. They eat like crazy, so therefore they poop inside you and this nasty stuff gets in your blood, your lymph, everywhere, even your brain. Now you know why you feel so sluggish and tired all the time. These toxins have an adverse effect on your central nervous system. Get cranky and irritable a lot? Ever wonder why?

Yes, the worms are disgusting, but the parasites you should be really worried about are the single-celled amoebas that get into your brain and organs.

Did you know that liver flukes can lead to cancer? You usually don't even know you have them, until of course you have so many, it's hard to avoid the symptoms.

Do you kiss or sleep with pets? Does your butt itch? Do you love bread, sweets and carbs? Do you eat sushi, or have you in the past ?

You got 'em!

Many times there are no symptoms at all. They can be in you for years until one day...

SIGNS YOU HAVE PARASITES:

- lethargy, feeling tired all the time (chronic fatigue)
- depression, forgetfulness, lack of focus, foggy thinking
- strong cravings for greasy foods and sugary foods, lots of carbs and bread, fruit, fruit juices, or alcohol
- eating more than normal but still feeling hungry
- digestive problems such as gas, bloating, constipation, or diarrhea that come and go but never really clear up
- irritable bowel syndrome (IBS)
- burning sensation in the stomach
- anemia or iron deficiency - worms can create enough blood loss to cause anemia or iron deficiency
- difficulty in losing or gaining weight, no matter how you try
- joint pain, muscle pain, and arthritis-like symptoms - pain in the back, shoulders, and thighs
- skin ailments such as hives, rashes, weeping eczema, itchy dermatitis,

acne, ulcers, sores, lesions, inflammation or swelling
- allergic-like reactions with no apparent cause
- itchiness in ears, nose, and anus
- excessive number of bacterial or viral infections
- candida yeast infection keeps coming back
- bleeding gums
- headaches
- restlessness or anxiety, nervousness; waste products from parasites irritate the nervous system, resulting in anxiety and restlessness
- fast heartbeat, heart pain
- insomnia, multiple awakenings during the night (particularly between 2 and 3am)
- teeth grinding and drooling during sleep, restlessness, dark circles under the eyes
- transmandibular jaw syndrome (TMJ)
- low immune system - parasites depress the immune system
- constant coughs and colds
- food allergies, food sensitivities, environmental intolerance or over-sensitivity (to smoke, chemicals, perfumes, etc.)
- loss of appetite
- sexual dysfunction in men - menstrual cycle problems in women

SOME TYPES OF PARASITES AND WHAT THEY DO:

Roundworms can lay 300,000 eggs a day! Over a million people are infected. Symptoms are upper abdominal discomfort, asthma, insomnia, appendicitis, peritonitis, and rashes due to the secretions or waste products from the worms. Large numbers can cause blockages in the intestinal tract, hemorrhaging (bleeding) when penetrating the intestinal wall, abscesses in the liver, hemorrhagic pancreatitis, loss of appetite, and insufficient absorption of digested foods. Adult worms grow to 15 inches/38cm long and look just like long spaghetti noodles.

Hookworm larvae penetrate the skin. When hookworms reach adulthood, they can sap their host's strength, vitality and overall well-being. Young worms use their teeth to burrow through the intestinal wall and feed on your blood. Symptoms from hookworm are iron deficiency, abdominal pain, loss of appetite, protein deficiency, dry skin and hair, skin irritations, edema, distended abdomen, mental dullness, and eventually cardiac failure (yes you can die from this!).

Pinworms infect one in five children. Symptoms are itching and irritation of the anus or vagina, digestive disorders, insomnia, irritability or nervousness. Female worms crawl out of the anus and lay about 15,000 eggs per day. Once airborne, the eggs can survive about two days anywhere in your living environment. Worldwide, about 500 million people are infected with pinworms. The worm is white and can grow to about half an inch in length.

Whipworm infections are estimated at several hundred million worldwide. Symptoms of whipworms are bloody stools, pain in the lower abdomen, weight loss, rectal prolapse, nausea and anemia. Hemorrhage can occur when worms penetrate the intestinal wall and bacterial infections usually follow. 1 to 2 inches length.

Amoebae are microorganisms that infect the end of the smaller intestine and colon. They release an enzyme that causes ulcers or abscesses where they can enter the bloodstream. They can eventually reach other organs like the brain or liver.

Trichomonas vaginalis are pathogens that resides in the vagina in females and the urethra, epididymis, and swelling in the prostate gland in males. In women there is some yellowish discharge accompanied by itching and burning.

Tapeworms may grow to 35 feet long and live ten years inside a person's intestines. Some tapeworms can lay as many as one million eggs per day. Their bodies are in separate segments with hooks and suction cups on their skull.

Flukes; Flatworms are found in bladder, blood, liver, lung, kidney and intestines. Human infections of flukes are in excess of 250 million worldwide. They can cause severe disease of the gastrointestinal tract, bladder, liver and destroy blood cells. Size varies from 1 to 2.5 centimeters in length (1/2 to 3 inches long).

Spirochetes are very tiny organisms that are spiral-shaped, and multiply in the blood and lymphatic system. Spirochetes (largest), Saprospira, Cristispira, Treponema (smallest), and many more. The host or carrier is usually lice, ticks, fleas, mites, and flying insects, which then transmit the organisms to humans. Most people's mouths are filled with Spirochetes, because they love sugar, bread and junk food. Bleeding gums is a good sign you have them. Once in the bloodstream, they make their way to the heart. Spirochetes are connected with heart disease, relapsing fever, infectious jaundice, Lyme disease, sores, ulcers, Vincent angina and Wyles disease.

THESE ARE JUST A FEW! THERE ARE THOUSANDS OF TYPES OF PARASITES. *YOU HAVE AT LEAST SOME OF THEM, GUARANTEED* !

Some parasite worms have the ability to fool bodies into thinking they are a normal part of the tissue or organ and the immune system will not fight off the intruders. When these alien invaders are established in our bodies, they do several things: they can make Swiss cheese out of your organs. Worm infections can cause physical trauma by perforating (burrowing) the intestines, the circulatory system, the lungs, the liver or the whole body.

They rob us of our vital vitamin and mineral nutrients, and amino acids needed for digestion. People become anemic and are drowsy after meals. Parasites poop toxic wastes that poison our bodies. They depress the immune system, which leads to further degeneration, fatigue and illness. They can destroy cells faster than cells can be regenerated. Some conditions that promote parasitic infections are excess mucus, an imbalance in the intestinal flora, chronic constipation, and toxic internal environment.

Humans with worm infections may feel bloated, tired or hungry, allergies, asthma, gas, digestive disorders, unclear thinking or toxicity. Some people may not have any symptoms from infection.
By the way, parasites LOVE bread, pasta, chocolate, agave nectar, fruit, carbs and other sweets as much as you do :-)

Whatever you like, they like. Whatever you don't, they don't. In other words, they love sweet stuff and hate bitter stuff. This is what makes things tricky and this is how they survive.

Also get rid of stress and human parasites in your life, work on relationships etc. External parasites attract internal parasites.

HELP!!! HOW DO YOU GET RID OF THEM?

SIMPLY TRYING TO KILL THEM RIGHT AWAY WON'T DO ANY GOOD, for two reasons. Firstly, they are in multiple stages - you might kill the adults, but not the half million eggs deposited throughout your body. These things are designed to survive. Secondly, think of parasites as your garbage men. Their job is to eat up your garbage. If you kill them, the garbage in your body will just keep accumulating until you die of over-toxification. The first thing you do is CLEAN UP YOUR BODY, which takes away their food supply. Stop eating all that modern processed food, especially bread, pasta, pizza, sugar and baked stuff. As a matter of fact, it's best to stop eating at all and do nothing but a month long juice fast, along with LOTS of colonics to help clean out all that gunk from your bowels. As you do so, the parasites will start freaking out and release chemicals into your bloodstream that make you CRAVE that bad food. But DON'T give it to them! Starve those buggers!!!!
It's either you or them. Then when you are clean and they are weak, THAT'S when you hit them with everything you've got - the strong herbs that knock them out and make them leave your body. You need to make

your body SO clean and spotless that they have NOTHING to eat and then flooding your body with parasite-ridding herbs will weaken, kill and flush them out of you like crazy. Unless you are really bad off, you won't see whole parasites coming out because after killing them, your digestive system starts digesting them. You might be pooping half digested parasite bits. Then you also have to hit the larvae and eggs in phase two. This is not a simple one week thing - this takes months and months - so you need to make this a LIFESTYLE.

There isn't one thing that will kill all parasites. The best thing is to go on a fast and starve them of their food supply, then hit them with a combination of plant-based, all natural parasite-killing herbs. I developed one that has the top most powerful herbs. You can get it at ParasiteFree.net. If you can't do a fast, then at least take the herbs and stop eating stuff that the parasites like. Do enemas or colonics to flush them out. Also do lots of (non-fruit) juices - cucumber juice is really good - worms HATE that stuff because it contains the enzyme erepsin, which digests the proteins of tapeworms... and remember to drink lots of water and do plenty of colonics to flush them out.

Parasites are everywhere. You cannot avoid contact. They are on all surfaces and even in the air. The only defense is having a super clean body that is well oxygenated with a strong immune system and a CLEAN digestive tract. If you eat comfort food, you are breeding parasites. MUCUS is a perfect breeding ground for bacteria and parasites. What causes mucus? Processed cooked modern foods, breads, cheese, alcohol, milk, dairy, stress, and anything not naturally found in nature. Mucus is the body's way of protecting your delicate tissues, but that warm gooey mucus is a perfect breeding ground for parasites. So keep clean!

AVOID ALL MEATS, DAIRY, SWEETS, JUNK FOODS

It's time you became aware what was going on inside you. "Out of sight - out of mind" is no good. What you don't know will catch up to you. Educate yourself on true health. Drugs are NOT the answer because they kill both good and bad bacteria inside you, and there is no single drug that kills all kinds of bacteria and parasites. Drugs are toxic poisons... you need a safe natural formula with MANY kinds of herbs that kill different parasites. The ONLY answer is to make yourself CLEAN right now and start respecting your body and never again feeding the aliens with junk and processed food... because if you don't, they will outnumber you and win. It's YOU or THEM. Starve them out, then kill them with PARASITE-FREE when they are weak.

The older the worms, the longer it takes to kill them. Just like people; the older they get, the stronger their system becomes and can deal with a lot more harsh contact. Persistence is the key and eventually nothing can withstand the onslaught of powerful herbs or medicine, over and over.

You can help get rid of parasites with simple household stuff.

The best program is to do a **Liquid FAST**- lots of vegetable juices like green leafy stuff, celery, cucumber, ginger, garlic. The more bitter the better. Or if you are up to it, do a two week fast with lemon water.

You will never get rid of all parasites. Many of them are necessary- they are little "garbage men" cleaning up our junk inside. The trouble begins when we eat too much garbage and they multiply like crazy. If there is nothing for them to eat, they either go to sleep or leave your body. They don't like clean healthy bodies. They love mucus and junk food. If you don't respect your body, the parasites wake up and start "recycling" your body, so only healthy people can continue the human species. This is nature's grand design. Eat right, stay clean and live long. It's real simple. Those who stray from nature's design pay the price.

Don't consume anything that feeds parasites - make them weak - starve them out and they'll leave on their own. Do not eat anything sweet, no breads, dairy, meat, rice, pasta, cereal or anything made from wheat or flour. Only raw stuff.

Second, do colonics or **Enemas**... you need to wash them out as they weaken.

My friend's wife did nothing but a juice fast and passed entire nests of worms! They wanted out of that body and left on their own. Bitter green juices really help, like dandelion juice.

Eat lots of fresh **Garlic**. Garlic is able to slow and kill over sixty types of fungus and twenty types of bacteria, as well as some of the most potent viruses. Garlic has a history of killing parasites and controlling secondary fungal infections, detoxifying while gently stimulating elimination, and has antioxidant properties to protect against oxidation caused by parasite toxins. The active components in garlic that kill parasites are allicin and ajoene. These compounds can kill amoebas, including one-cell varieties, as well as pinworms and hookworms. Allicin is not present in garlic in its natural state. When garlic is chopped or otherwise damaged, the enzyme alliinase acts on the chemical alliin, converting it into allicin, the active component contributing for its success at killing parasites. Use crushed or juiced garlic for serious power.

Lots of cucumbers - they contain enzymes that kill tapeworms.

Green Papaya - full of protein-dissolving enzymes (parasites are protein) and especially eat the peppercorn-like papaya SEEDS - they are powerful.

Watermelon (with seeds) - the seeds contain powerful stuff.

Clove - cloves contain the most powerful germicidal agent in the herbal kingdom, known as eugenol. They also contain caryophyllene, which is a powerful antimicrobial agent. These components travel through the bloodstream, killing microscopic parasites and parasitic larvae and eggs. Cloves are tremendously effective in killing malaria, tuberculosis, cholera, scabies and other parasites, viruses, bacteria and fungi, including

103

candida. Cloves also destroy all species of shigella, staphylococcus, and streptococcus.

Raw Pumpkin Seeds - able to kill eggs, contain a natural fat that is toxic to parasite eggs. Curcurbitin in pumpkin seeds has shown anti-parasitic activity, since it has the ability to paralyze worms, leaving them to drop off the intestinal walls. Chinese scientists used pumpkin seeds to treat acute schistosomiasis and tapeworm infestations. Many parasite formulas contain pumpkin seeds, but they don't do much in just a few capsules. You need half a cup 3X a day to really work. Grind in a coffee grinder and add to salads, smoothies, soups and so on.

Nutmeg - also contains eugenol, a powerful killer of parasite larvae and eggs.

Turmeric - powerful cancer-fighting, anti-inflammatory, wound healing, worm-expelling body purifier.

Cayenne - destroys fungus, mold & parasites on contact. Increases circulation and health. Increases effectiveness of other herbs.

Ginger - increases circulation and helps all digestive issues, also good for relieving gas and nausea associated with parasite die-off.

Take **ENZYMES** containing large amounts of **protease** (which digests protein and parasites; bacteria and viruses are protein).
Do not take if you have a bleeding digestive system or ulcers. Enzymes shouldn't be for long term use or your body will stop making it's own.

Take **probiotics** at the end of each day, at least 8-10 hours after taking parasite herbs because those killing herbs knock out everything, including good bacteria.

Scrub your hands, keep fingernails clean, wash all produce, pet owners wear slippers, practice impeccable hygiene.

More things that help get rid of parasites:
- **Hot peppers**
- **Onion**
- **Lots of green tart apples** (not store-bought apple juice - that's sugar. It's the pectin-fiber of the apples that does the work.)
- **Wild spicy greens, like mustard greens**
- **Fennel seed**
- **Oregano oil**
- **Olive leaf extract**
- **Grapefruit seed extract**
- **Aloe Vera**
- **Colloidal silver**
- **Thyme**
- **Una De Gato (Cat's Claw)**
- **Myrrh**
- **Bitter melon** is effective against pinworms.
Fasting on nothing but **raw pineapples** for a week helps with tapeworms.

Take some sort of fiber during your cleanse, also colon cleansing is recommended to flush out the dead parasites. My parasite formula already has colon herbs in it, but most people need more push. Use my **COLON-FREE** formula.

Remember- they love sweet stuff and hate bitter stuff, just like you. That's why they can live inside you so easily. Let this be motivation to get off the sweet stuff, which makes you fat anyway, and put more bitter things in your diet, which cleans the liver. The liver is where your body gets its energy, hormones, interferon and many other things, so more bitter! It makes parasites leave and look for food elsewhere.

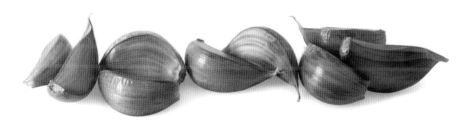

PARASITE-KILLING HERBS:

(These are the herbs in my PARASITE-FREE formula, which can be ordered at **ParasiteFree.net** Do not take if pregnant or nursing.)

Note: Couples should both do a parasite cleanse at the same time, otherwise they just re-infect each other.

Green Hulls of Black Walnut: shown to have powerful effects on killing many varieties of parasites. The dried and ground green hulls of the Black Walnut contain tannin, which is organic iodine, as well as juglandin. Black Walnut has been used for centuries to expel various types of worms, including parasites that cause skin irritations such as ringworm. It oxygenates the blood, which also helps kill parasites. Black Walnut is very effective against tapeworms, pinworms, Candida albicans (yeast infections) and malaria. It is also effective in reducing blood sugar levels, and helping the body rid itself of toxins.

Graviola Bark: is a major component used in my formula because of the amazing results for purging parasites. Graviola has a great record of killing intestinal parasites, calming nerves, reducing blood pressure and helping arthritis, heart and liver: Some people saw parasites in their toilets after just one day of using this stuff! Graviola has been researched in laboratory tests since the 1970s, where it's been shown to: effectively target and kill malignant cells in twelve different types of cancer, including colon, breast, prostrate, lung and pancreatic cancer... 10,000 times stronger in killing colon cancer cells than Adriamycin (a commonly used chemotherapeutic drug). REFERENCE: http://www.greenwoodhealth. net/np/graviola.htm. Graviola contains the chemical annonaceous acetogenins, this is the active compound that is harmful to parasites.

Quassia: a tree native to Jamaica and its neighboring islands, has traditionally been used as a remedy for roundworms and as an insecticide. It has also been used as a bitter digestive aid and a remedy for digestive disorders, parasites, and head lice. See naturalstandard.com .

Butternut Bark: used specifically for parasite cleansing. Butternut is a native of the midwestern and northeastern United States and has been used since the 1800s as a laxative and in the elimination of parasites. Butternut is also used to support healthy liver function. Butternut, also called White Walnut, is used to expel, rather than kill, worms (vermifuge).

Wormwood: named for its ability to expel parasites, this bitter herb is known worldwide for its strong killing ability. This is one of the MOST POWERFUL tools in the parasite-killing herb kingdom. It is most effective against roundworms, hookworms, whipworms and pinworms. Wormwood contains the potent chemicals thujone and isothujone, which are the primary components that kill parasites. Wormwood also contains santonin, an effective remedy for parasitic diseases. Wormwood is the second most bitter herb known to man and has been proven as a POWERFUL remedy for malaria. Wormwood also contains sesquiterpene lactones, which work similarly to peroxide, by weakening the parasites' membranes, therefore killing them. Wormwood also helps produce bile, which in turn helps the liver and gallbladder.

Oregon Grape Root: contains berberine, a substance known to kill most forms of bacteria, viruses, fungus & parasites.

Diatomaceous Earth: food grade version is used as a parasite "shredder". Diatoms act like glass passing over skin, cutting the fragile flesh of all living adult parasites on contact (without harming humans). It is also a dessicant, meaning it dries out anything fluid, so it goes inside the parasites' shells and dries up their insides. Can be used on humans and pets. If you dust it on the floor, it keeps ants and bugs away. Also a great source of organic silica for hair, nails and skin.

Olive Leaf: mentioned in the Bible, along with the olive fruit; "the olive fruit shall be as meat, and the leaf as medicine." Current research shows the leaf is anti-bacterial, fungal, viral, microbial & parasitical.

Rhubarb: used to help expel the die-off of parasites, eggs and larvae. We chose rhubarb as it is not addictive like other colon movement stimulants, and is very powerful, even in a low dosage.

Cloves: contain the most powerful germicidal agent in the herbal kingdom, known as eugenol. They also contain caryophyllene, which is a powerful antimicrobial agent. These components travel through the bloodstream, killing microscopic parasites and parasitic larvae and eggs. Cloves are tremendously effective in killing malaria, tuberculosis, cholera, scabies and other parasites, viruses, bacteria and fungi, including candida. Cloves also destroy all species of shigella, staphylococcus, and streptococcus.

Pumpkin Seeds: able to kill eggs, contain a natural fat that is toxic to parasite eggs. Curcurbitin in pumpkin seeds has shown anti-parasitic activity, since it has the ability to paralyze worms, leaving them to drop off the intestinal walls. Chinese scientists used pumpkin seeds to treat acute schistosomiasis and tapeworm infestations.

Red Raspberry Seed (Ellagitannin): raspberry seeds usually pass through our bodies, but when ground up, they contain one of the most powerful antioxidants known: Ellagitannin (Ellagic Acid). Aside from being used very successfully in cancer treatment, Ellagitannin has also been found to be a powerful destroyer of parasites. It's a very strong anti-bacterial, anti-fungal, anti-viral that lowers cholesterol and protects our DNA. This stuff is very expensive and hard to get, but worth every molecule.

Aloe Vera: this plant, called "herb of immortality" by the Egyptians, contains a soothing gel that helps peristalsis. Aloe Vera has antibacterial and anti-fungal activities. Aloe destroys bacteria more powerfully than any other hypoallergenic plant known.

Papain: papain is a protein digestive enzyme that really works synergistically with herbs to further break down material. This digestive enzyme will help restore your intestinal tract to its normal state, which makes it inhospitable to parasites. Papain taken thirty minutes before or after meals helps kill worms.

Cat's Claw: this herb is often used for treating stomach ulcers, gastritis, eczema, "break-bone fever," and liver diseases. Since the 1980s, Cat's Claw has most commonly been used in modern herbal medicine as an immune stimulant. The oxindole alkaloids in Cat's Claw strengthen the immune system and also improve circulation, by lowering blood pressure. The master rain forest herbalist Leslie Taylor has used Cat's Claw tinctures and teas to treat cancer and HIV with remarkable success.

Goats Rue: is a wild legume used during the Middle Ages to treat the plague. It was also used to induce sweating to break fevers and to treat infections from parasitic worms and snakebites. This herb can help balance blood sugar levels, help women balance hormones and the plant has no odor, unless a stem or leaf is bruised, causing the release of a stench, hence the name "Goat's Rue." Effective in both humans and animals alike.

Garlic: is able to slow and kill over sixty types of fungus and twenty types of bacteria, as well as some of the most potent viruses. Garlic has a history of killing parasites and controlling secondary fungal infections, detoxifying while gently stimulating elimination, and has antioxidant properties to protect against oxidation caused by parasite toxins. The active components in garlic that kill parasites are allicin and ajoene. These compounds can kill amoebas, including one-cell varieties, as well as pinworms and hookworms. Allicin is not present in garlic in its natural state. When garlic is chopped or otherwise damaged, the enzyme alliinase acts on the chemical alliin, converting it into allicin, the active component contributing for its success at killing parasites.

African Cayenne: 120k HU is the most powerful variety of cayenne pepper, able to destroy fungus, mold & parasites on contact.

All parasites are bothered by different things, so it helps to take a large variety of things. This is why our product contains so many different types of herbs, because its just too hard to really kill all different types of parasites with simply a few different herbs. I would also recommend grinding Cloves in a coffee grinder to add to teas, salads or smoothies.

BLEEDING GUMS: a serious warning sign

Gum disease is connected with heart attacks. People with periodontal disease are three times more likely to have a heart attack than people with healthy gums. Toxic bacteria enter the bloodstream, reach the heart and scar the arteries. Toxins and inflammation created by periodontal bacteria get into the blood stream and trigger the liver to release a substance called C-Reactive Protein (CRP), the levels of which, believe it or not, are a much more accurate way of predicting heart attacks than cholesterol levels. This CRP also leads to blocked arteries, blood clots, high blood pressure, sudden heart attacks, doubled levels of colon cancer, Alzheimer's, and all kinds of chronic serious immune problems. Have your CRP levels checked! If you have sensitive or bleeding gums, go to the dentist and have them cleaned NOW. Then STOP eating processed baked, cooked sugary carbs and animal products. Wash your mouth out with hydrogen peroxide and make your own tooth powder with baking soda, cayenne and sea salt. Floss, or even better, use a WATER PIC. Clean your blood and liver with a serious fast, herbs and colon cleansing. This is serious. Do not take bleeding gums lightly.

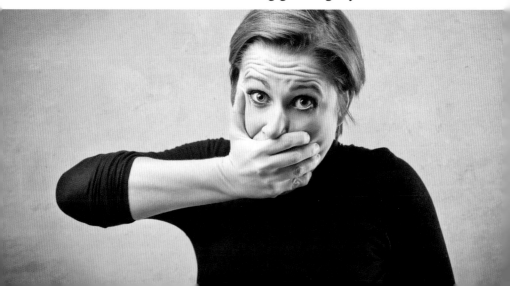

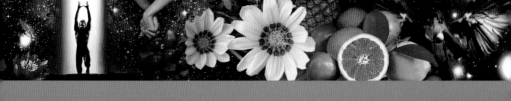

The Life-Changing Health Plan

WATCH THE MIRACLES HAPPEN

1. Do an enema or colonic every other day for at least a month. If you're really sick, do a number of enemas every day. Take large amounts of probiotics at the beginning and end of each day, to replenish intestinal flora (the good bacteria).

2. Stop eating solid food for a while. No, you won't waste away. This step is important. (Note: if you are on prescription medication, consult your doctor first. Chances are though that they won't want you to stop eating solids, because many drugs require food in your stomach and also doctors are not familiar with this centuries-old method of natural healing. Some drugs require food, so get off the drugs first)

3. Nothing but water for AT LEAST two days. As much water as you want. At least a gallon a day. This is called FASTING and it's mentioned in every religion and historical healing text around the world. Go as long as you can on nothing but water. Do a week or two if you can (make sure you are off medication by this point, otherwise jump to juice fasting). So the sequence is water, then vegetable juice, **then blended drinks and finally raw food.**

Every single day of the fast, do these things (including all-water days, juice days and blender days):

- Mornings upon rising, squeeze lemon juice (and lime if you want) into a glass of water and again late afternoon.

- 20 minutes later, two tablespoons of raw apple cider vinegar in a glass of water.

- enema or colonic at least every other day (time of day doesn't matter).

- walk outside in fresh air and sunlight for thirty minutes if possible.

- green or white tea, mornings and night (no juices after dark - just water and tea).

- fresh green vegetable juices during the day between 12 and 6 - as much as you want. (not on water-only days)

- in the afternoon, do another water with apple cider vinegar or lemon.

- add magnesium and MSM to your water throughout the day.

- stretch or do yoga stretching (see end of book for diagrams).

- if you have a mini trampoline (rebounder), use it 15 minutes a day.
If you don't have one, jump up and down anyway. Also play inspirational music and dance every day when no one is around. It's time to open your soul and body.

- breathe really long and deep, filling your lungs all day with air as much as you can.

- remain in a relaxed state of being. Nothing bothers you any more.

- tell people you love them.

- stay close to home. You are in reclusive introversion mode. The caterpillar must seal itself into a cocoon in order to come out as a butterfly.

- no television, no news. The world will do fine without you during this time. Insulate yourself from anything potentially depressing... news, people, etc. Only listen to soft, inspirational healing music. If you don't have any, buy some relaxation CDs.

- take long hot baths with apple cider vinegar or Epsom Salts in the bath water (available at any drugstore, even grocery stores). Turn the lights low. Light some candles, play soft music. Drift away. Sweating is good. Fall asleep if you want. You are a baby in the womb again.

- be asleep by 9 or 10 pm. No exceptions. Healing hormones are released between 10pm and 2am and you must be asleep to receive their benefits. Every hour of sleep before midnight adds to your health, while every hour of sleep lost after 10 pm takes away from your health.

EXAMPLES OF JUICE DRINKS

(It's a good idea to have celery in everything - it's one of the most healing foods, very high in electrolytes. Ginger is a miracle food also - especially for digestion and circulation. Add garlic to everything if you have illness.)

celery, cucumber, apple, parsley

celery, cucumber, carrot, spinach, ginger

celery, cucumber, ginger, apple

celery, cucumber, beet, spinach, ginger, garlic

celery, watercress, carrot, ginger

celery, beet greens, carrot greens, ginger

celery, parsley, dandelion, carrot, ginger

celery, cucumber, kale, apple, garlic

celery, cucumber, garlic, lemon

cucumber, beet greens, blueberries, lemon

celery, cucumber, grapes, lemon

celery, watercress, lemon

celery, kale, apple, ginger, garlic, lemon

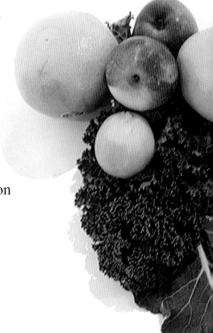

Don't juice sweet fruits; the sugar will be too concentrated and feed candida, viruses, bacteria, yeast, mold and parasites. Tart green apples are OK.

If you have cleaned all of the toxic crud out of your body and your cells, your intestines and colon are clean, and the only thing you are putting in your body is water, fresh vegetable juices (especially greens with lots of chlorophyll) and some herbs, then you are forcing foreign viruses, bacteria, cancer etc to be in an environment in which they cannot exist.

HOW LONG TO STAY ON A JUICE FAST

Stay on the juice fast as long as you possibly can. Every day you go longer, the deeper the healing will be. Some people feel so great after a month that they go for a second and third month. You might not see or feel what's going on, but trust me - there is a LOT going on inside you, on a deep cellular level. You can't clear out thirty or forty years of bad living in just a matter of days, or even weeks. The more time you give it, the more fine-tuning your body can do.

Do NOT let peer pressure stop you short. Remember, you will be detoxing and just like a house during spring cleaning, you might look like a mess, and if people see you they will probably say you need to stop this "unhealthy" thing you are doing and that you are "wasting away". You are only wasting away the years of bad living. Like an exorcism, you might look like crap during this time. Do NOT let people scare you into stopping. Stay strong and listen to the inner you! Shoot for a month, especially if you have a serious condition. If not, go for at least a week or two. The food cravings will end after a few days and you will hit a beautiful smoothness, like when airplanes hit 30,000 feet and there is no more turbulence - just beautiful open sky. At this point it becomes a spiritual experience. You will feel so wonderfully high and calm. Give your body all the time it needs to clear away a lifetime of bad habits. Your liver is bigger than your head and it is filled with decades of toxic goo - it will take time to clear it all out. But the payoff is a new, longer, healthier life, like you never experienced before.

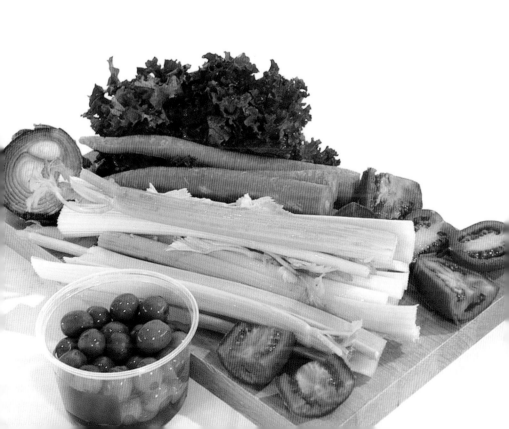

STEP 2: BLENDED DRINKS

Then, move on to blended drinks. NO SOLID FOOD YET!!!!! But this is a step in that direction. In this phase, you are moving from juicer to blender, and consuming the whole fruits and vegetables - pulp, fiber and everything... just in a liquified state, so it's already "digested" for you, saving your body lots of energy. In terms of using the "whole" food, a watermelon with seeds and rind is OK, but obviously do not put a whole peach in the blender with the pit. If you have any of my supplements, now is when to start adding them. (not the water or juice phase, except maybe the parasite formula)

The basic rule is to use **at least half leafy green**s and half (or less) fruit in each blended drink. Do NOT blend just fruit - that's too much sugar. The secret healing stuff is the leafy greens. Yeah I know, that's not the part you like, but that's what works the miracles. Hey, at least you are introducing some fruit in there. Be thankful.

Blended drinks are a complete food. They contain everything you need for life and you can live on them indefinitely. You are consuming the whole fruits and vegetables, just like you would find them in nature... you are just liquifying them first before swallowing, which saves your body a lot of work in terms of digestion. This also solves the assimilation problem that most salad-eaters have. You get a lot more nutrition and calories from blended drinks than if you just ate it. We need to consume two good-sized bunches of dark leafy greens a day. This doesn't sound very appetizing I know - so that's why we have the Vitamix blender! The magic trick is to simply add some fruit with the greens; liquify it all, then just drink it down. Voila. Health :-) It's important to still "chew" it though, because this releases needed pre-digestive enzymes. It's also important NOT TO CHUG it down. Sip it slowly over half an hour- so it takes just as long to consume as if your were eating all that stuff in a bowl. This is important. if you find yourself hungry later, it means you swallowed it too fast. You should not be hungry after a smoothie because there are more calories absorbed than just eating.

You might find, like others have, that after consuming green smoothies every day, your moles, warts and skin blemishes simply fall off one day. People have even mentioned cancer scabs peeling off in the shower, leaving healthy new skin underneath.

Green leafy vegetables have almost all the amino acids, minerals, enzymes and phytonutrients we need... the trouble is they're locked into cells made out of cellulose, which is really tough. In order to get to the nutrients, the cellulose needs to be broken open and that requires a LOT of serious chewing and that's why cows and horses chew all day long. That's also one of the reasons they get so big. We hardly chew our food and our stomach acid is normally nowhere near strong enough to digest the cellulose, therefore the nutritional value of the green plant foods we eat is hardly ever utilized and that's why so many vegetarian/vegan/raw foodists are so skinny - they aren't assimilating their nutrients. This is also why they get grey hair and wrinkles - they are malnourished even though they are eating the right food. The secrets are: 1 - they need stronger stomach acid and 2 - they need to break their food apart more, either by chewing until their food is creamy liquid goo, or BLENDING their salads! And guess what, when you consume a lot of green smoothies (especially with bitter greens), your stomach acid gets stronger again, like it's supposed to be! Remember- bitter is better. Bitter stuff helps digestion, cleans the liver, helps skin, hormones, improves mood, helps depression and immunity, whereas sugar leads to depression, lowered immunity and weak energy.

You can test to see if your stomach acid is strong enough by drinking some beet juice and if your pee or poop turns color, then your stomach acid is too weak. That's why you have gas and health issues. Also, since stomach acid is supposed to kill parasites in our food, most people have parasite infestations because of the weak acid. As a matter of fact, many parasites breed in our stomachs and intestines like crazy because that's where all the food is. Weak stomach acid and parasites can lead to almost any health condition you can think of.

In the meantime, to jump start the stomach acid, take HCL pills and put apple cider vinegar in water two times a day and salad dressing. Also take TMG (trimethylglycine) 1000mg 3x a day. Don't worry, it's made from beet roots. Also take 50 mg zinc once a day with food and my herbal vitamin C (needed for stomach acid) and my green formula because it has really high levels of B vitamins, also needed for stomach acid. You could take a B vitamin pill, but many of those are synthetically made.

If you are worried about food combining between leafy greens and fruit, don't worry - leafy greens are NOT vegetables and can be mixed with anything (and they should be). Do NOT mix carrots, beets and other roots with fruit. Those are starches. BUT carrot and beet greens (tops) are OK! As a matter of fact, we have it all backwards - we should consume the green tops more than the starchy roots. The greens have hundreds of times more vitamins than the bottom part, which is mainly minerals & starch. If you want serious Vitamin A, blend the carrot tops, not the root part.

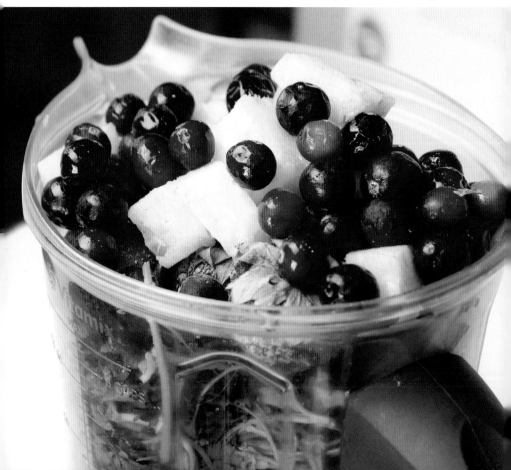

EXAMPLES OF GREEN SMOOTHIES (liquid salads)

Note*: each smoothie must include at least half green leafy material like kale, romaine, parsley, celery, spinach, dandelion etc. The chorophyll (what makes it green) is needed for the magic to work.

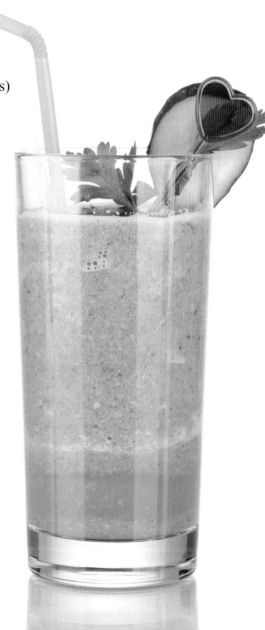

1 bunch of spinach or kale
2 cups of papaya
2 cups water

_____

1 bunch spinach or kale
2 peaches or nectarines(no seeds)
2 cups water

_____

1 cucumber
3 pieces celery
1 bunch spinach
2 tomatoes
lemon juice

_____

6 leaves kale
1 banana
mango
piece of Aloe Vera
2 cups water

_____

head of romaine/kale
strawberries
frozen banana
2 cups water

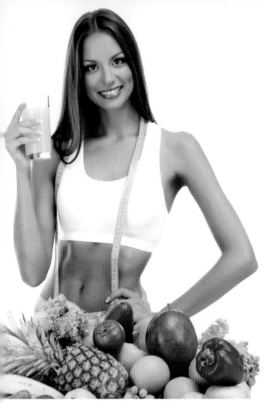

romaine
celery
cucumber
blueberries
1 or 2 dates
piece of Aloe Vera
coconut water

You get the idea:
half green leafy stuff
half fruit
and some liquid.

Avoid carrot, beet, parsley root (green tops are OK), during serious cleansing.

Remember: keep doing those enemas or colonics and end the day with lots of probiotics (liquid non-dairy form is best).

You can add 1 or 2 dates for sweetness. They are high in fiber and fiber helps slow the aborption rate of sugar into the body.

While you are cleansing, make sure to get enough rest and sleep, otherwise you will be defeating the purpose. Stop eating at 6 and be asleep by 9 or 10.

After a week or two of blending, or however long you can last... or once you know for sure that you are healed, you can reintroduce solid food. Make sure it is RAW, uncooked food... the more moist the better - use high water-content items like juicy fruits and vegetables. Minimize nuts, seeds and dehydrated stuff in the beginning.

Always have at least one green smoothie every day, preferably for the rest of your life :-)

RAW FOOD

Finally here we are. Solid food. Ahhh.
OK. Don't go nuts. Take it easy. Start with soft stuff.

Always try to stay with juicy, wet foods as much as possible - like fruits and other things that are the way you would find them if picking them off a tree or bush in nature. In other words, apples and watercress are more natural than dehydrated crackers or raw cheesecake made out of cashews. Those don't grow on trees in nature. They're ok, but don't go crazy with sweet stuff, you don't want to ruin all that hard work. Sea vegetables are a great salty addition to anything plus they have iodine for thyroid which helps regulate weight.

Grinding your own flax seeds into powder in a coffee grinder is much better than buying flax meal or flax crackers, but only grind what you need as you need it, to preserve as much life force as possible. The same goes for anything ground up or juiced or blended. Make your food yourself as much as possible and consume as soon as possible after making it.

Do NOT juice fruits and then drink the fruit juice straight without watering it down 50% first - the sugar concentration is too strong for our bodies, which causes too much of a glycemic spike in the blood. It also feeds pathogens (viruses, bacteria, mold, yeast, fungus and ulcers). It's always best to combine fruit with some kind of green leafies. In the wild, animals eat just as much leaves as fruit in combination.

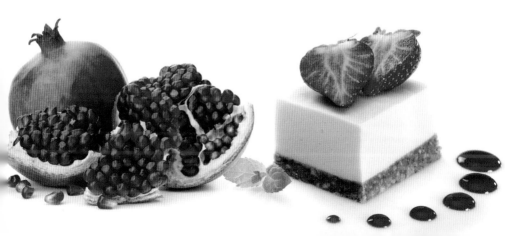

Eat fruit by itself, or with green leafies is OK, but nothing else. No soy milk, no granola, no yogurt.

Don't mix fruits and vegetables (leafy greens don't count as vegetables). Lemon, lime and tart apples are OK.

Wait a few hours after a meal before eating any fruit. Fruit digests very fast and if other food is still in your stomach, the fruit will ferment it, causing the whole mess to go bad and cause gas. Not a pretty picture.

If you possibly can, get fruit right off the tree or bush, when it is fully ripe. Most fruit in a grocery store is picked un-ripe, and they can never ripen like they are supposed to because there are no more nutrients coming through the branch from the mother plant. Unripe fruits are not good for us because they are not ready to eat.

TRANSITIONAL FOOD: SWITCHING TO RAW

What most people consider "raw" food isn't really raw living food. The healthiest food is food that still has life in it - meaning if you planted it in the ground, it would grow (and I don't mean mold). For example, plant a tomato or apple and you get a tomato or apple plant growing out of the ground. Plant a pumpkin seed and pumpkin grows. Most people miss the addictive, traditional sweet carb foods they grew up on, so they want to eat food that tastes like hamburgers, bread, cheesecake, crackers, coffee, chocolate, cookies, pies... and they spend a lot of effort mimicking those tastes and textures with raw food. And that's OK. Whatever it takes to go in the direction of health. And there are some VERY tasty cheesecakes that taste exactly like or even better than real cheesecake. Instead of using dairy products, they are made with things like cashew nuts, coconut oil and so on. The crust is made with ground up nuts mixed with dates for example. But once something is ground up into a paste or powder, it is no longer alive. It will still have its vitality for a while, but eventually oxidation sets in and after a few days it is bland dead food. These foods should be eaten the same day they are made. It's still better though than eating that store-bought commercial processed crap full of chemicals, preservatives, bad trans-fats and poisons.

So if you need to, then eat the transitional foods - like dehydrated crackers, burgers, cookies and so on. But just know that it's not as health-promoting as fresh fruits and vegetables plucked right off a tree, bush or vine and eaten whole or blended. You might not be able to pick your own food in this modern world, but at least buy what you can at the local farmers' market or grocery store, and then just eat it with minimal preparation. For example, you can simply slice up some strawberries and bananas in a bowl, sprinkle some cinnamon on top and voila: breakfast. For lunch, throw some celery, mango and kale in a blender with some water and voila: lunch! Have a salad in the middle of the day with some apple cider vinegar and hemp oil. Chop a few dates in there if you want. For dinner, have a bowl of papaya with lemon juice. Eat the seeds too. See where I'm going with this? This is almost as simple as an animal in the wild eats, except with a bit of human touch.

It's also very simple, easy to do and doesn't take a lot of time. And that's very important in this day and age. Food should not take up a lot of our day. It should give us energy, NOT make us feel tired afterwards, NOT lead to health problems, not give us gas, and not weight us down or slow us down in any way. It should make us feel great, keep us going all day long with no highs or lows, go through us in a matter of hours and come out with no problem or smell.

Raw chocolate and raw cheesecake are what I consider occasional feel-good snacks, but are not part of my everyday diet. When people come over, it's a nice way to celebrate, make friends and pull people over to healthy living by showing them how good stuff can taste. I have included some recipes later in this book. But when I am alone, I really don't put a lot of energy or thought into food. Preparing food seems like such an inconvenience to me; I want to create art, play, make love and travel the world. There is too much to do in this world to be slowed down by worrying all the time about breakfast, lunch and dinner.

STAY CLOSE TO NATURE IN THE FOOD YOU EAT

While you are on a healing diet cleanse, I seriously suggest you stay away from dehydrated raw foods and all of those desserts, cakes, pies, burgers, chocolates and so on, until you are well. Stick to things the way they are found in nature... LOTS OF LEAFY GREENS and juicy fruits and vegetables and maybe occasionally a few soaked seeds (seeds are better than nuts). Do not mix seeds with fruit unless they are part of the fruit. Green leafy matter is where the magic healing power is. Blending is the best way to consume this green magic. The recipes in this book are healing.

POWDER VS. FRESH

There are times when fresh fruit is not as nutritious as powdered fruit. This is because moisture is an oxidant, which means the moment something is picked, it starts to oxidize and lose vitality. Within a few hours, half the vitamins may be gone. One test showed a number of grocery store oranges had no vitamin C left at all. Zero. If however you were to instantly dry and powder the plant, it's nutrients could stay intact for years. This is why I sell powdered plants and why its important for YOU to eat freshly picked plant foods and not let them sit on the shelf for a week. This may be difficult for many city people, but just be aware of this. Do what you can.

FIBER

Almost everyone in the modern world is seriously deficient in fiber. Tests show 97% of Americans don't even meet the minimum recommended daily amount. Animal products have zero fiber. Fiber does a lot more than just push things through the digestive system. It helps slow down the sugar release into the blood and helps clean out our bodies, acting like a sponge soaking up toxic crap inside us, including estrogens and heavy metals. Fiber is also the main food source for our gut probiotics, which is basically 75% of our immune system and regulates our metabolism and weight. Insufficient or weak gut flora leads to everything from diabetes to autism, obesity, autoimmune disease, IBS, Crohns and eventually life threatening disease. Fiber is absolutely necessary for health, especially those with sugar issues. Fiber is so important to our well-being and health. It is the reason why blended drinks are better than juiced (although juices are good for stage one of healing anything, when the body can't handle fiber). Flax crackers are common fare among raw foodists, but to me they often taste like dried cardboard and may be hard on the body. Remember, everything has to be turned into liquid blood inside us and we also don't chew our food like we are supposed to (it's supposed to be a creamy liquid goo with no chunks when we swallow it). Flax is good for you but the seeds should be ground in a coffee grinder first or else they just go right through you without doing anything. After grinding, put in water, salads or smoothies. Great source of EFA Omega oils and of course, fiber.

Chia seeds are even better than flax and not as hard on the body because they turn into a jelly goo after 5 minutes in water. They are a great source of fiber, protein and EFAs (essential fatty acids) - you know - the Omega oils. AND fiber AND B Vitamins. Simply put a couple spoonfuls of chia in water and drink... or you can blend it in a blender first. Chia seeds are one of the best sources of EFAs and they are easily digestible. Did I mention they are a source of protein? :-)

SEEDS and NUTS

are designed by plants to be eaten by animals, carried somewhere else and then pooped out, so that they can grow into new plants. They are small so that they can be swallowed whole and they are coated with enzyme inhibitors so that they won't be digested by stomach acid. This coating is acid-proof but is dissolved away by water. This is so that the seed or nut can survive the trip through an animal's digestive system, and then when the seed or nut is laying on the ground again in a pile of poop (aka fertilizer), it sits there patiently waiting until it rains. Presto! The protective coating is dissolved and the seed or nut instantly starts to sprout. Yes, this is fascinating trivia, but what does that have to do with you? Well I'm trying to explain why you can't just pop seeds and nuts in your mouth and expect to get a lot of nutritional value from them. They will probably just irritate your stomach and intestines.... UNLESS you soak them in water overnight... ah... then the magic elixirs of life are made available to us. By the way, seeds are better for us than nuts. In the wild, chimpanzees don't touch nuts but they occasionally eat seeds. Did you know almonds are a seed, not a nut? Chimps also don't eat roots (carrots, beets, etc) but they eat the greens on top of these roots, and of course, the fruit. Take a hint. My suggestion is when on a healing, cleansing diet, eat only stuff from above the ground, and later on you can eat the starches.

MINERALS
Minerals are necessary for 95% of your life-sustaining functions. Unfortunately, today's soils are so depleted of most of the stuff we need that the plants grown in them are deficient also, therefore we need minerals from somewhere else. The best source is SEA VEGETABLES. Consume about 2-3 spoonfuls of sea vegetables each day. Take scissors and snip them into your salads and soups or just throw some in your blended smoothies like I do. A great taste combination is the saltiness from seaweed mixed with the acidic sweetness of pineapple. My green formula is a convenient quick source of minerals and vitamins.

VARIETY*** ROTATE WHAT YOU EAT
We need to rotate what we eat, and as great a variety as possible. Each plant has certain nutrients that are different from other plants. If we keep eating only the same fifteen things, no matter how healthy they are, we will develop deficiencies and have health issues. The more types of foods you eat, the more chance you will be getting what you need, nutritionally. This is another mistake that many raw foodists make: they keep buying the same fruits and vegetables that they like and after a while they develop a deficiency and wonder why. Rotate. Variety is the spice of life!

As a general rule:
JUICER - greens, vegetables and non-sweet fruit.
BLENDER - use any combination of fruits and greens.
Basically, only put fruit in a blender, not a juicer. You need the fiber to buffer the high sugar content of the fruit. Most fruit is so soft and juicy - just EAT the dang thing!

You can also put a handful of grass in the blender with your smoothies. Nothing wrong with that. You get ALL the fiber, phytonutrients, minerals, vitamins and co-factors. Just make sure you drink this concoction within ten minutes or else it starts oxidizing, loses its value and it also begins to taste funky.

Apple Cider Vinegar, HCL pills and TMG and zinc to jump start your stomach acid (do the beet juice test to check your HCL level).

At night, take liquid non-dairy probiotics before bed and also mornings.

THE PLAN

Method 1: Overnight

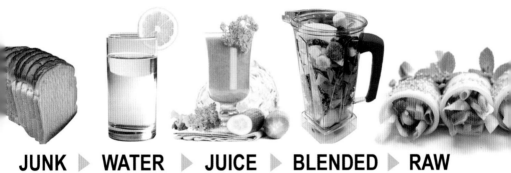

JUNK ▶ WATER ▶ JUICE ▶ BLENDED ▶ RAW

Method 2: Easing In

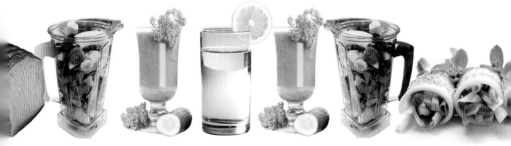

IK ▶ BLENDED ▶ JUICE ▶ WATER ▶ JUICE ▶ BLENDED ▶ RAW

SAMPLE DAILY MEALS

I really don't have "meals". I don't have a schedule. I eat when I'm hungry and I don't when I'm not. If I don't eat for half a day I don't care, because I know that's healthy - it's called fasting. Just make sure that you drink enough water or juice and you'll be healthy, happy and full of energy. I only drink water until noon, but most people can't do that right away, so here is a more user-friendly daily plan.

Upon waking: large glass of water, sometimes with fresh lemon juice

BREAKFAST - Always keep it light; you are "breaking the fast" you just had all night. Here are some Examples:

-papaya with lemon juice and garlic (also eat as many of the papaya seeds as you can)

or

-strawberries and banana slices with cinnamon on top

or

-smoothie (in blender) - strawberries, frozen cherries & cranberries with different kinds of leafy greens and lemon juice, green formula herbal vitamin C two cups water

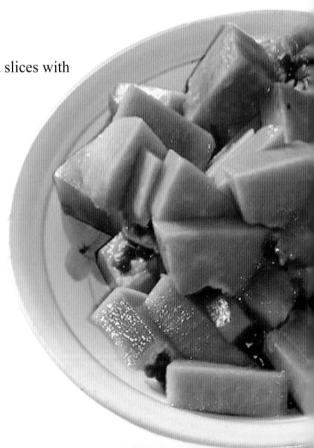

Sample breakfast drink 1:
2 fresh Aloe Vera leaves
2 oranges
1 grapefruit
1 lime
1/3 cabbage
1 cup fresh pineapple
1/2 cup tocotrienols
1 cup water
3 tablespoons my green formula

Sample breakfast drink 2:
2 Aloe Vera leaves
coconut water and meat
1 cup cranberries
1 bok choy
2 dates
2 tablespoons herbs
2 stalks celery
16 oz water

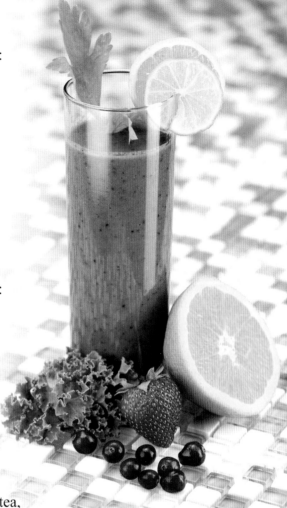

Mid Morning - white or green tea,
or glass of water with 4 tablespoons tocotrienols (rice bran solubles) or
chia seeds, or
bowl of durian blended with coconut water/meat with strawberries on top.

I go to the gym late morning so that I can have lunch right afterwards
(biggest meal).

LUNCH - (biggest meal of day) - see my recipe section on the next page
or any meal from any raw food book. Some ideas are:
-one of the meal recipes pictured on the following pages.
-raw soup (blender) -carrot juice, avocado, ginger, garlic, celery, cayenne
-simple salad like arugula, red onions, hemp oil, lemon, apple cider
vinegar, nutritional yeast, black pepper, touch of sea salt.

Mid Afternoon

Green smoothie (half fruit, half leafy greens) - see GREEN SMOOTHIE recipe ideas.

Example: celery, pineapple, mango, kale, kelp, water

Late Afternoon

Raw food snack, like dehydrated dandelion bread topped with apple sauce (simply blend 2 apples).

or

Enjoy two bananas.

or

handful of Marcona almonds and sea salt.

DINNER

(done eating by 6:30)

One of the meal recipes on the following pages

If you absolutely need to have a cooked meal, then have one for dinner to celebrate your good behavior throughout the day. Be sure to take TMG and some HCL pills beforehand. No meat, bread, pasta, wheat, dairy or cheese. Just be aware cooked meals are not optimal and create fat quicker.

Early Evening

Optimally, you should STOP EATING BY 6:30 pm! No more snacks, smoothies or even juice. Just tea or water. But if you really need something while transitioning, then drink a glass of water with 4 tablespoons tocotrienols (rice bran solubles) and chia seeds.

or

papaya with lemon

Evening - Water with probiotics, magnesium and (optional) night formula.

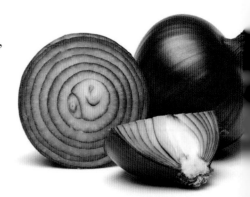

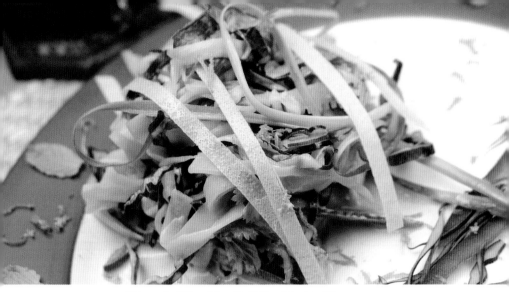

RECIPES

It's pretty simple. Buy everything that looks good in the grocery produce section (bitter stuff too!) and just throw stuff together when you're hungry. Everyone's taste is different. Listen to your body - it will tell you what it needs. Just remember to have lots of dark leafy greens every day... and believe it or not they go with everything. I put kale and sometimes even grass in my morning fruit smoothie and it tastes great. Don't overdo the sweet stuff, even natural sugar - everything in balance.

Anyway, here are some samples of what I eat with pictures and ingredient lists. These are actual pictures of stuff I personally made just before I actually ate it :-) I don't have a lot of time, so these are all recipes that I can throw together quickly. I just use anything I have laying around. Coconut water is the sweet liquid base for my smoothie concoctions. Since there's no cooking, I just put everything right into a bowl and eat! Forget calling it "main course" or "dessert" - with raw food, everything can be your main course - even fruit. Use this as a starting point to whatever works for you. After that you can get our Uncookbook "Love on a Plate" which has easy to make healthy versions of your favorite dishes like pasta, pizza, chocolate cake, creme brulee, mac n cheese and a lot more. In the mean time, grab whatever looks good and throw it in a bowl. Have fun!

MANGO BLUEBERRY MINT

recipe video at MangoGarlic.com

mango
blueberries
fresh mint leaves
chopped jalapeno pepper
tiny bit of chopped garlic
fresh chopped ginger
juice of 1 lime
sea salt

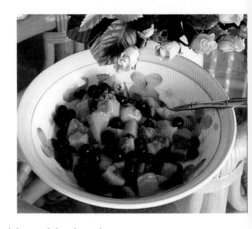

This mixture tastes amazing even without blueberries.

DURIAN CUSTARD PUDDING

recipe video at DurianRecipe.com

In blender:
durian & coconut water / meat
(mainly all durian)
vanilla
bit of lemon juice
top with fruit - MMMMmm !!!!

Most of my meals are just stuff
lying around thrown in my Vitamix
Blender.

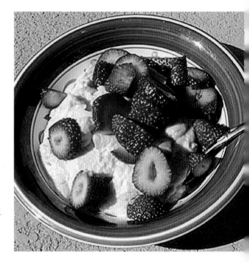

QUICK VITAMIX MEAL

video at AwesomeBreakfast.com

coconut (water and meat)
red leaf lettuce and/or kale
seaweed
pineapple
asparagus
parsley
fresh sprouts
celery

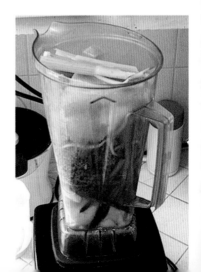

KALE SALAD

2-3 bunches kale
chopped onion
cucumber
lots of black pepper
dash of sea salt
1/3 cup olive oil
1/3 cup apple cider vinegar
1/3 cup fresh orange juice
2 tablesp nama shoyu (raw soy sauce)

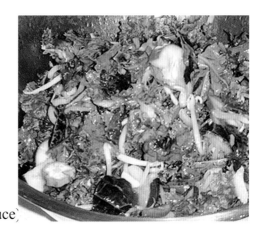

AVOCADO TROPICAL SALSA

video TropicalSalsa.com

avocado
papaya
mango
red onion
olive oil
apple cider vinegar
cilantro
sea salt
black pepper

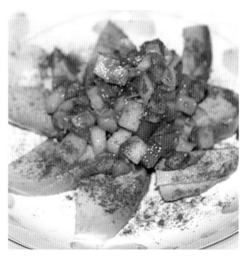

SPICY THAI CABBAGE

video SpicyThaiCabbage.com

red cabbage
raw cashews
scallions
cilantro
raisins, sea salt
raw nut butter
apple cider vinegar
hot chili oil
sesame oil
sea salt

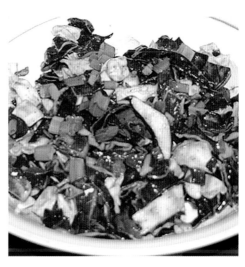

SILICA SALAD

(Silica is good for skin, bones, joints, hair, teeth, lungs etc)
red leaf lettuce, cucumber, okra
nopales (cactus), red onion
Dressing: orange juice, nama shoyu, olive oil.
Spiced Nuts - shake nuts in bag with raw honey, sea salt, cayenne.
Note: put the okra and cactus in just before you eat. Their high silica content makes them slimy after an hour - that's natural and OK.

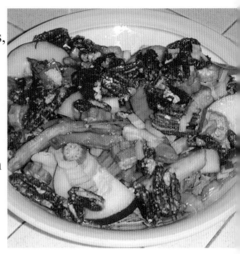

RAW FRUIT PIE

Raw fruit pies are now available at most health food stores. This one is from "Go Raw" here in Las Vegas. (I added more fruit). These are NOT cooked/baked, all ingredients are raw and just mixed together.
blueberries, coconut oil, cashews
agave nectar, lemon juice,vanilla
sea salt
The crust is ground nuts & dates.

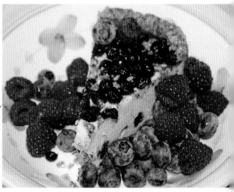

SUPER FAST GREEN BLENDER MEAL

coconut water
avocado
red leaf lettuce
parsley
sea salt
(cashews on top)

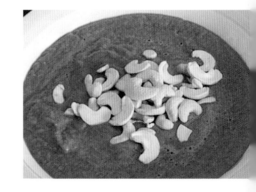

FAVA BEANS

video FavaBeanRecipe.com
Fava beans are great for anti-aging
growth hormones and male prostate
support.

fresh raw fava beans
olive oil
minced garlic
minced hot pepper
touch of apple cider vinegar
sea salt

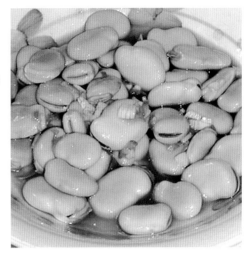

KALE FUN SALAD

Again, mix whatever you want with
kale.This one has:
tomatoes, sprouts, cucumber,
red leaf lettuce, mustard greens
onions, cilantro, garlic, radishes
sea salt, sauerkraut, date pieces

Dressing: equal parts of fresh orange
juice, nama shoyu, olive oil.

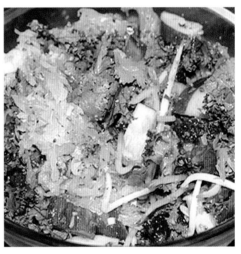

DECO CABBAGE SALAD

red decorative curly cabbage
red or orange bell peppers
cucumber
basil
oregano or cilantro or parsley
chopped garlic

Dressing: olive oil, apple cider
vinegar, nama shoyu.

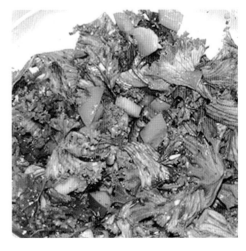

RAW CHOCOLATE TREATS

RAW CHOCOLATE "MILK"

In Vitamix blender:

12 cacao beans

meat and juice of 1 coconut

7 raw cashews

1 big tablespoon coconut oil

3 teapsoons maple syrup

cinnamon

pinch sea salt

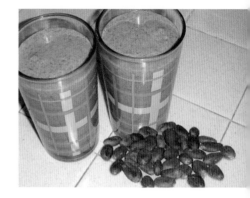

RAW CHOCOLATE

video at FreezerChocolate.com

(see next page for recipe)

cacao beans

raw carob powder

raw nut butter

maple syrup or agave nectar

coconut oil

peppermint oil

vanilla

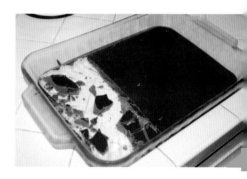

Simply grind beans into powder, mix with the other ingredients and leave it to chill.

INGREDIENTS FOR MAKING RAW CHOCOLAT

8 oz RAW Carob powder

1oz Vanilla
(non alcohol) or real vanilla bean seeds

2 oz Peppermint flavor

16 oz extra virgin unprocessed coconut oil

36 oz Raw Cholocate beans (Cacao nibs)

16 oz RAW Nut Butter of choice (cashew is smoothest)

6 oz Maple S Agave

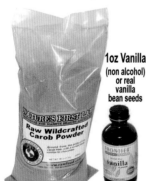

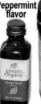

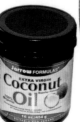

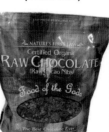

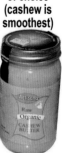

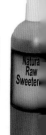

THE EXACT, STEP-BY-STEP RECIPE IS ON THE NEXT PAGE...

Yes this stuff isn't cheap, but it makes a lot. This should be enough for a month if you consider it a treat and not your main course. You can get all of this shipped to you from online sources, but this is becoming so popular, many health food stores are starting to carry this stuff too. Look closely though, the bigger chain stores like Whole Foods have ROASTED carob powder (not raw) and most nut butters are not raw, so read the labels. I use peppermint and vanilla oils that don't have alcohol as a base. Try not to use oils in an alcohol base for this.

Coconut oil comes in different grades - make sure you get the raw extra virgin untreated, unheated kind. It's usually a tiny bit more expensive. Coconut oil is clear like water at room temperature, but when it's colder, it gets white and hard like wax. It become liquid again inside your body, unlike hydrogenated oils used in commercial chocolate.

The steps are pretty basic. The main thing is to grind the cacao nibs (chocolate beans) into a fine powder. I use a standard little coffee grinder. The raw chocolate is so rich with natural oils that it will stick a bit to the grinder, so you'll have to use your fingers to scoop it out. The rest is basically mixing it all together with a wooden spoon until it's smooth. That's it. There is NO cooking, baking or heating. You can mix it together and eat it right then and there while it's like chocolate soup, but I like it hardened, so I put it in the freezer and break pieces off when I want some.

's a great way to lure unhealthy people to the healthy side :-)

So , raw food is not just carrot sticks and celery :-)

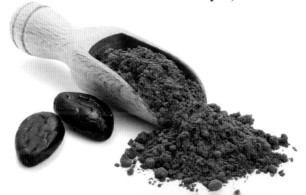

Note: if cleansing from serious illness, wait with chocolate until you are better because of the sweetener. Stay as clean as possible when cleansing.

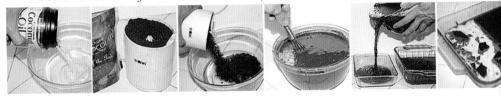

HERE ARE THE CHOCOLATE-MAKING STEPS...

1. Pour coconut oil into a bowl. If the oil is hard, warm it in the sun or in hot water first until it's clear liquid. A little heat won't hurt it. MAKE SURE IT'S CLEAR LIKE WATER.

2. Grind the cacao nibs into a fine powder (in a coffee grinder).

3. Add the cacao powder to the oil, along with all the other ingredients.

4. Stir until all the lumps are gone.

5. Pour the mixture into shallow pans. I like to keep it at around half an inch thickness.

Put the chocolate pan(s) in the freezer and in about ten minutes the chocolate is hard and ready. Break into pieces and ENJOY!
Cacao is pure dark chocolate. It's where chocolate comes from. If you are European and love dark chocolate, you can eat the beans right out of the bag if you want, but for most people it's a little too strong and bitter, s that's why the carob is mixed in - to mellow out the bitterness. Everythin here can be altered to taste. It's really hard to make bad chocolate. The cool thing about raw chocolate is that if you screw up, you can always fix it. For example, when I think it's too sweet, I simply set it on the counter at room temperature - it becomes liquid again in about thirty minutes and I just mix in more cacao and carob, or maybe some more nut butter - you get the idea. You can just keep changing it! Raw is so cool because ther is no "point of no return", unlike when you're cooking.

TIP: the type of nut butter you use makes a difference. Make sure it's RAW and organic. The best kind is by ARTISANA and my favorite by far is RAW CASHEW butter, not just because of the flavor but because it's CREAMY like butter and makes the chocolate really silky smooth. Almond butter is supposed to be the healthiest but it's grittier and may cause your chocolate to be a bit rougher in texture. Artisana nut butters are available in health food stores or can be ordered online via internet.

TIP 2: make sure the carob powder is RAW, not roasted. It usually has clumps in it, so be sure to break those apart with your fingers before mixing everything else in.

You need to keep the chocolate in the freezer and if you take any pieces out, you need to eat them right away, because the oils start to melt at room temperature. This is the difference between good oils and bad oils (good chocolate and bad chocolate). If it's made to keep for a long time at room temperature, it has saturated fat/hydrogenated oils, which are very bad for you. I like to put macadamia nuts in the mixture, so that I have crunchy bits to bite into. Enjoy !

See the video of me making the chocolate at **FreezerChocolate.com**

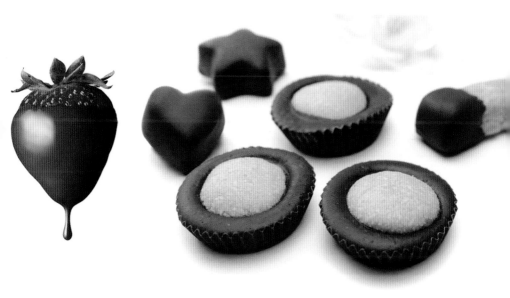

SIGNS OF DETOX AND LEVEL OF HEALTH

How can you tell if you are better, or still getting rid of bad stuff? Energy level and mood are both great places to start. If you are popping out of bed at the first rays of sunlight, 6am, going going going all day long with no drop in energy, and you don't need a lot of sleep and you mood is up all the time with no depression, then you are on the road to health. If your energy isn't what it used to be when you were a kid, you aren't healthy yet. No matter how old you are. There are 80 year olds with energy levels that would do circles around most.

Most people don't know that mood and emotion are also big signs of health. Even if you have money and relationship problems, it won't bother you as much because mood is a chemical thing and if the chemicals in your body are right, you can handle almost anything. Sure, something might knock you down for a minute or a few hours, but you bounce right back with overwhelming optimism and a sense of universal peace. People will wonder how you can remain so calm while the rest of the world could be falling apart around you.

Another sign to gauge your recovery is how slimy your mouth and tongue is in the morning when you wake up. If your throat and tongue are coated with mucus or have a white filmy coating on it, you are still detoxing. You still have things in you that are making your body grow yeast and fungus. The body creates mucus to protect you from stuff. These things could be foods, chemicals or even just stress.

How you smell: when you have become totally clean, you will have no more bad breath or body odor and your pee and poop won't smell anymore. If they do, something is still rotting and detoxing inside you. Another sign of health is that you need less and less food to do the same amount of work. This means that your body is becoming more efficient and assimilating nutrients. People who are hungry all the time and need to keep eating are that way because they aren't getting proper nutrition absorbed into their system from their food. It doesn't necessarily mean that they are eating the wrong food, it just means their bodies can't draw the nutrients from that food - either because they aren't digesting the food properly (low stomach acid, not chewing enough, stress), or their intestines are lined with mucus and plaque which won't allow nutrients through. Most people have both problems.

The only way to start absorbing nutrients is to get the intestines clean again. This means a month's worth of serious colon cleansing with enemas, fiber, probiotics and herbs. That's why I created my FREE-COLON and CHARCONITE products... to help clean things out. Charconite is charcoal and bentonite - the two most powerful absorbers of bad stuff - mixed with herbs to help move it through. Free-Colon is a great source of natural, non-irritating fiber and bioflavonoids, which not only help the digestive tract but also help clean the cardiovascular system. My Prebiotic Fiber helps feed the gut flora and flourish.

If you have a headache or pain anywhere in the body, you have a blockage. Something is blocking something. Do enemas/colonics, stretching exercises, drink lots of water and do emotional cleansing.

Remember: YOU WILL GET WORSE BEFORE YOU GET BETTER. Your body will strip down to bare bones and start over. You WILL lose weight. Most of it is water (held in your body by all that salt) and fat which is where the toxins are stored) You will most likely smell bad, break out with zits, get weak, tired, look anemic, get headaches, get congested, your lungs will fill with mucus, your nose will run like Niagara Falls, your kidneys will hurt and you will probably get cold and flu-like symptoms. You will want to curl up in bed and just sleep. People will mock you and tell you to end this silly stupid health kick thing. They will say "See? You look terrible. It doesn't work, come on, eat some real food" and other stupid demoralizing comments like that. Just know that this is detoxing. Forty years of soft drinks, cheese and pizza do not get flushed out of your cells in a week. This takes time. You will even have old problems flushed to the surface - afflictions you had years ago, like childhood allergies, rashes, possibly even old fears etc. Your body is doing SERIOUS spring cleaning. Old thoughts and emotions might even surface. Again, don't freak out - just know what's happening. Look at the hell that detoxing cocaine addicts go through. Or cigarette smokers. You always thought you were better than them, didn't you? Ha! We're all in this together. Nobody is immune to being human. Our issues are just different, that's all. This really makes you appreciate what the other people have to go through. If you don't think you're an addict, JUST WAIT until the first time you try to not eat cheese or bread or anything with sugar for the first time (haha - evil laugh). As they say, you have to crawl through hell to make it to heaven.

Put it this way: If you eat right, you won't need a doctor. If you eat wrong, there's nothing they can do. Don't ignore your body's signals and warnings. Don't hide them with medication. If you have pain or discomfort, your body is trying to tell you something. If you simply keep doing what you've always been doing, you're just going to get worse.

Remember to do a liver cleanse and enemas/colonics during this phase, or your liver will clog up from all that sudden waste being dumped.

To keep yourself going, just know that others have made it through and like grubs that became butterflies, they became new people. Don't just take my word for it - read as many books and internet articles as you can about other people who did this and how their problems went away. Nothing is free, everything has a price, and this one definitely is worth it. Like Tonya Zavasta says, don't do it for your health, do it for your vanity. Do it so that you can be amazingly sexy and attractive.

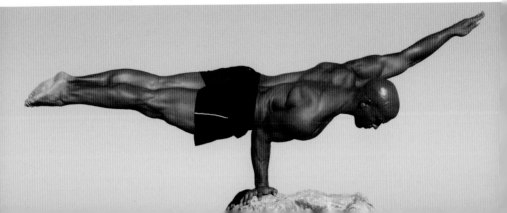

MISTAKES MANY RAW FOODISTS MAKE:

- too many SWEET and dessert foods - like fruit juice, chocolate, "raw" cheesecake, cookies, cakes, parfaits.

- too much fruit , not enough greens and BITTER stuff

- too many dehydrated foods - crackers, cereal, breads, kale chips, candied nuts.

- not enough cleaning out** (enemas/colonics) to help detox regularly (one of the biggest). People skip enemas but need to do them

- not enough leafy greens (should be half of diet - second biggest reason for issues is not enough greens).

- roots should not be main "vegetable" source -starches are hard on the body when not cooked. Save these until after you are better

- don't chew food enough (undigested cellulose, causing gas, malnutrition).

- not enough stomach acid (from too much sweet stuff, not enough bitter, stress, lack of sleep), hence the gas.

- don't exercise enough * - cardio and weight bearing exercises are necessities.

- bad food combining (nuts with fruit, etc).

- too many ingredients in recipes - keep things simple.

- don't soak nuts and seeds

- too many nuts (seeds are much better).

- eat before bed (should stop eating after dark, 3 hrs before bed).

- agave nectar (see number one). At least use MarkusSugar.com

- eating the same foods over and over - not enough variety leads to deficiencies).

stress (too worried about things) or **in denial** (head in the clouds, not grounded).

not enough vital minerals (seaweed, magnesium, MSM etc).

don't go to sleep early enough (around 10pm at the latest).

didn't get mercury fillings removed - major toxic dump into body from raw detoxing.

cheating more than you think. It's OK until cheating becomes addiction.

BAD THINGS TO AVOID

Toothpaste, hair products, detergents with **Sodium Lauryl Sulfate**. This chemical can cause skin irritation, permanent eye damage (especially in children), skin rashes, hair loss, flaking skin and mouth ulcers. Easily penetrates skin and can lodge itself in the heart, lungs, liver and brain.

NEGATIVE PEOPLE. Get rid of them. They're bringing you down and suck your energy.

THE NEWS. It panders negativity and numbs your brain. You have better things to do with your life

MIDNIGHT MUNCHIES. Go to bed hungry. Your body needs a rest. Stop eating at 6 pm!

AVOID PLASTIC BOTTLES if you can - they contain estrogenic chemicals. Use glass - refill and reuse glass bottles.

If you heat a **nonstick pan**, and a bird is a few feet away, it will die from the toxic fumes.

STRESSFUL JOB. No excuses. This is only a test. Trust me.

CARPETS are a major source of synthetic fumes and major collectors of allergens and parasites.

BLEACH - replace with sodium percarbonate or hydrogen peroxide.

UNNATURAL LAUNDRY DETERGENT- all kinds of problems

Air **DRY CLEANED** clothing outside for a day.

MOBILE PHONES DAMAGE DNA, damaging even the next generation of cells. At least use speaker phone mode or earphone cord.

CHLORINE in drinking water causes scarring of the arteries and leads to artherosclerosis. Use a filter on your shower and kitchen. Hot showers create chlorine gas which knocks out thyroid leading to weight gain.

FLOURIDE is one of the most toxic chemicals in the world. It's more toxic than lead and only slightly less toxic than arsenic. It causes all kinds of diseases like thyroid, bone and brain cancer and leads to obesity and depression.

MICROWAVE OVENS - eating microwaved food causes lymphatic and thyroid disorders, cancer, leukemia etc. It poisons baby food and even just microwave-heated water. If you use microwaved water to water a seed, it won't grow.

Keep your distance from electric stuff as much as possible. Don't use electric blankets. If you live near high power lines, move, unless you want brain cancer. Minimize the low hum of air conditioners, computers, washing machines, dishwashers, car engines, etc - these frequencies affect every cell in the body and can throw them way off balance.

INDOOR LIGHTING. You need sunlight. It is pure life energy.

SYNTHETIC CLOTHING Go with cotton. It breathes.

FLORESCENT LIGHTING emits powerful damaging EMF

... did I say lose the negative people?

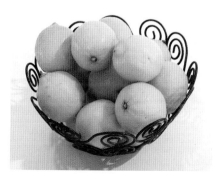

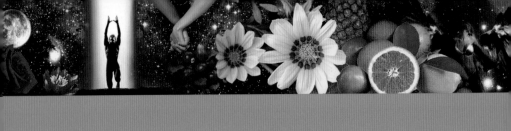

BODYWORK

MOVE IT OR LOSE IT!

'Anyone who lives a sedentary life and does not exercise, even if he eats good foods and takes care of himself according to proper medical principles--all his days will be painful ones and his strength shall wane."

(Maimonides, treatise of Hygiene 1199 A.D.)

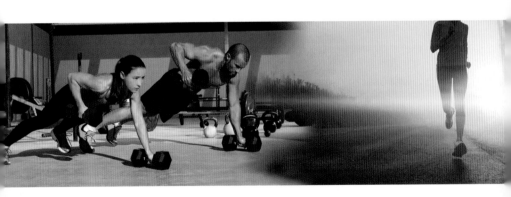

EXERCISE
MOVE YOUR BODY OR DIE

You can eat all the right food and still be unhealthy. Your body needs to move, there is no way around this. Just one day without exercise and your body parts start to atrophy and slowly die. Studies show a sedentary lifestyle has the same effect on heart disease risk as smoking a pack of cigarettes a day! We need some form of exercise every day. Exercise can turn back the clock 15-20 years! It's the best mood elevator of all. It reduces anxiety, relieves depression, and extends your life. Exercise is a must. Oxygen is more important than food. Moving you body is the ONLY thing that moves the lymph through your body and you have four times more lymph than blood. When you sit around all day, your trillions of cells are creating trillions of little cell poops and if you're not moving that stuff out, you become toxic and sluggish. Even if you are healthy and eat totally raw food, your cells are still pooping waste out every second and you need to keep that stuff moving out through your lymph, and exercise is the only way to do that. At least stand up every half hour and do jumping jacks or push-ups or something.

You have one body. Use it or lose it. Eyesight problems? Same thing. Eyes are muscles. You're probably not getting enough oxygen to your eyes (lack of exercise), and you probably spend most of your day in artificial light staring at a computer screen, paperwork, books and then go home and watch TV. Your eyes are made to look at things at a distance, and since you are not using those muscles you are losing your eyesight. Wearing glasses makes it worse. Do eye exercises and get your eyesight back!

Here's an exercise for those of you who feel you don't have much time for exercise - this just takes one minute - lie down on floor, stand up, lie down, stand up... as fast and as many as you can for one minute. Try it. You'll see what I mean! Do this every day.

WALK as much as you can!

Park your car as far from the entrance as possible. Take the stairs, not the escalator, and use every second step when you do. Get a mini-trampoline ("rebounder") and use it at least 10-15 minutes a day. It really gets lymph moving to eliminate toxins by stretching and squishing every cell in your body. Every cell in the body produces toxic waste. Every cell in the body needs stimulation in order for toxic waste to be eliminated (exercise!). Exercise is a must. Oxygen is more important than food. Try and walk/ run/jog outside in the fresh air and sunlight, not on a treadmill in a stuffy gym filled with recycled air from sweaty toxic people. People who live over 100 walk many miles a day every day. Climb stairs wherever you can. Don't take the elevator. Walk. Run. Jump. Skip. Swim. Roll around. Chase each other. Be fools. Swing from trees... I don't care: MOVE!!!!! And while you are at it - remember to BREATHE DEEPLY!

HOT AND COLD

This is so simple and yet so powerful. Basically you get your body real cold, then real hot, then real cold, then real hot, then real cold, and so on. What this does is make the blood rush to your skin and extremities to cool off when you are hot (skin turns red), and then when you are cold, the blood rushes to protect your inner organs (skin turns pale). What you are doing is causing a "pumping" action that forces your blood to hustle through your whole body, washing your cells as it goes. This is particularly good for anyone sedentary and people who can't move a lot - but it's powerful healing for ANYONE. The best way to do this is in the shower. Get as hot as you can for thirty seconds, then as cold as you can for thirty seconds, then hot again - do this half a dozen times. Scream if you have to. You will feel like a new, reborn person! Some people have done this to specific body parts and watched cysts and even cancer scabs fall off after repeated hot/cold therapies. Do it. No excuses!!!!

If you REALLY want some serious healing power, fill a bathtub with ice and sit in it for 15 minutes. I did a video on that.

STRETCH

This is SO important. Your muscles need to stretch; just like wringing out a wet towel, stretching your muscles squeezes your body's cells and forces the waste out, and then sucks nutrients and oxygen in. That's why we feel so enlivened and so much better after a good stretching set. And I don't mean just sitting in a chair, putting your arms behind your head and yawning. No, I mean getting up and touching your feet and stuff like that. I have included photographs and diagrams here to show you easy stretching exercises you NEED TO DO every day! If you are getting sore and stiff, this is why. When you sit motionless for hours on end every day, you are slowly dying. Part of the reason people have fat in their stomach area and butt is because when they sit, those areas get crunched and circulation is cut off. Good circulation is needed to remove fat from cells. Stretching helps get blood back into those compressed areas.

YOGA

No, this isn't some new age religious cult thing where you meditate and go OOOHM. It's basically a nice combination of stretching, exercise, breathing and de-stressing which helps loosen and strengthen your body, mind and soul. I used to think I didn't need this because I already went to the gym. Hah. A lot of those yoga exercises are TOUGH! They seem easy but wait till you try them. You'll be shaking within the first three minutes. They really open up your body in so many ways that are highly beneficial, yet most people aren't aware of this. Yoga helps energy flow through your body more. It helps release blockages and strengthens you... not just physically but mentally and spiritually too. If you are old and stiff, don't worry - this doesn't force you to do harmful or painful things. Do whatever you can and you will come out of it better than when you went in. These are just body movements - that's it - it's not an eastern religion class, don't worry. You don't need to do yoga in a class. You can easily do it at home. Better still, go outside and do yoga in nature. Come on folks - it's just a bunch of stretches and calming exercises. If you have a lot of stress in your life, this helps. Many of the following stretches (pictures) are considered as yoga postures.

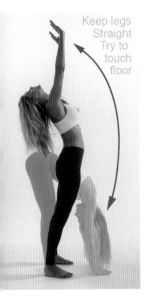

Keep legs Straight Try to touch floor

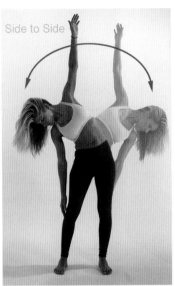

Side to Side

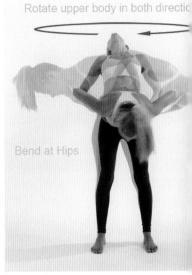

Rotate upper body in both directio

Bend at Hips

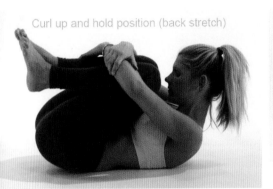

Curl up and hold position (back stretch)

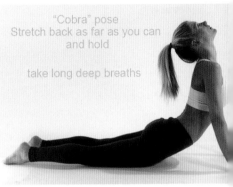

"Cobra" pose Stretch back as far as you can and hold

take long deep breaths

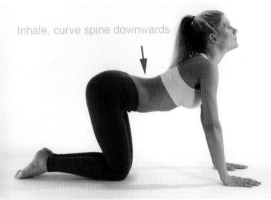

Inhale, curve spine downwards

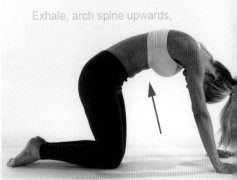

Exhale, arch spine upwards,

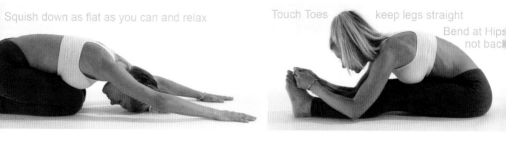

Squish down as flat as you can and relax

Touch Toes   keep legs straight
Bend at Hips
not back

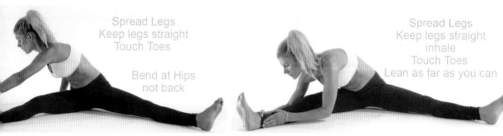

Spread Legs
Keep legs straight
Touch Toes

Bend at Hips
not back

Spread Legs
Keep legs straight
inhale
Touch Toes
Lean as far as you can

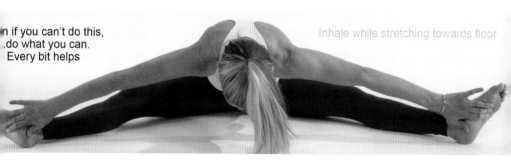

n if you can't do this,
.do what you can.
Every bit helps

Inhale while stretching towards floor

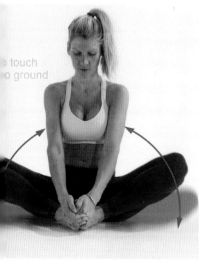

touch
o ground

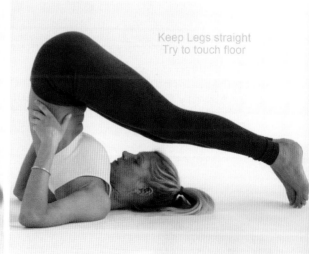

Keep Legs straight
Try to touch floor

151

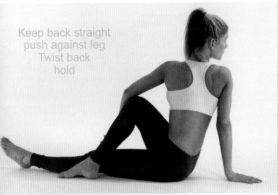

Keep back straight
push against leg
Twist back
hold

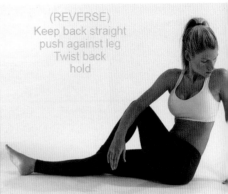

(REVERSE)
Keep back straight
push against leg
Twist back
hold

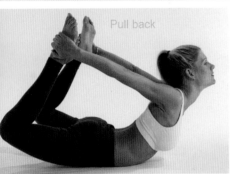

Pull back

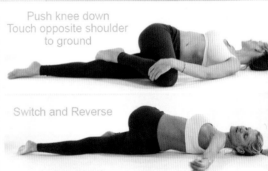

Push knee down
Touch opposite shoulder
to ground

Switch and Reverse

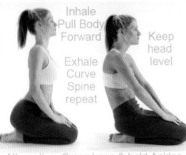

Inhale
Pull Body
Forward

Keep
head
level

Exhale
Curve
Spine
repeat

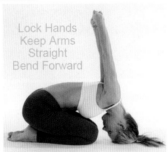

Lock Hands
Keep Arms
Straight
Bend Forward

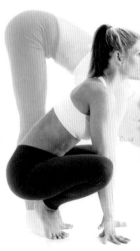

Alternative- Cross Legs & hold Ankles

These simple stretches are the basic core
of almost every health course worldwide.

Do these every day

It doesn't matter when

<u>Just do them</u> !

Try to keep heels off ground
Straighten Legs, inhale
Squat, exhale,
Repeat

Daily Stretching 1

RECOMMENDED HOUSEHOLD BODY DEVICES

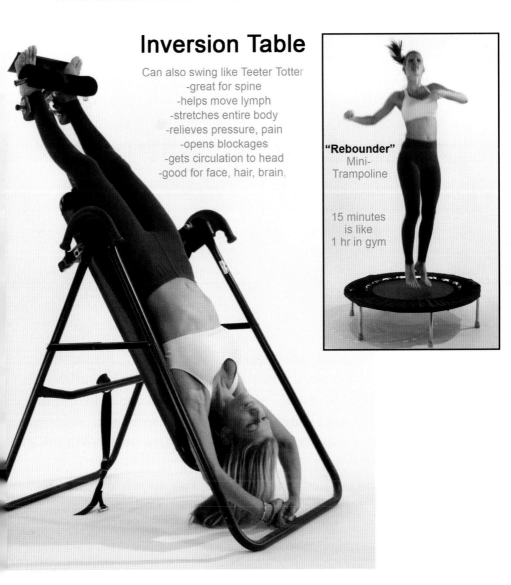

Inversion Table

Can also swing like Teeter Totter
-great for spine
-helps move lymph
-stretches entire body
-relieves pressure, pain
-opens blockages
-gets circulation to head
-good for face, hair, brain,

"Rebounder"
Mini-
Trampoline

15 minutes
is like
1 hr in gym

**These are a couple of gadgets I have in my human hampster cage.
Every hour or so I get up and use one.**

Daily Stretching 3

EMOTION, MIND & SOUL

The most important feeling in the world is being at peace with yourself.

Your body is just a reflection of how you feel inside. Feelings always affect your body and your body always affects your feelings. They are one. When we hide feelings our body suffers from ulcers, headaches, cancers, tumors and so on. Simply eating raw food isn't going to make you disease-proof. It sets the stage, but the actors you put on the stage determine the show. And those actors are your feelings.

New scientific tests are now showing beyond a shadow of a doubt that our feelings are more powerful than anything we have imagined. They can literally create our reality. It's called the field of Epigenetic Medicine, and a great book on the subject is "The Genie in Your Genes" by Dawson Church, Ph.D. I could write a book on this subject alone, but I'll try to sum it all up as briefly as I can.

Your cells are little soldiers waiting for instructions, and they are willing to go to war and die for you. Every single one of them. Just say the word. So watch what words you use. That is where you need to be careful. Because your cells don't understand sarcasm... they take everything that you say literally. For example, if you keep saying "I feel like shit and wish I could die", guess what, you start having bowel problems, turning into shit, and your body cells start to age and die. If you are heart broken, your heart starts to weaken. Many people have literally died from a broken heart. If you feel undesirable, your body actually starts making you undesirable. If you feel great and happy about your life, your body starts to miraculously heal, many times defying logical explanation. This process is instantaneous. Scientists have seen DNA change before their eyes within seconds of people's thoughts changing. In one test, a person's blood tested free of diabetes, then within minutes, when his personality changed, the blood was taken again and the person was found to have diabetes. Thoughts are the most powerful healers or killers in our lives.

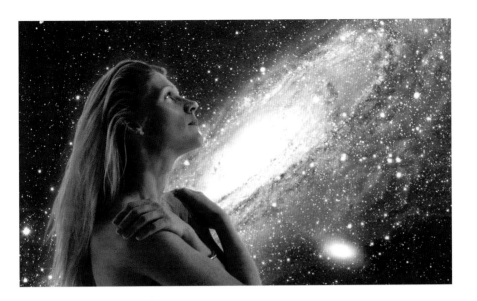

Every thought, every moment, every action, has a powerful impact on the cells of your body. Positive, high vibration thoughts can rid your body of disease. Negative, stressful, low vibration thoughts can give you disease. Be careful what you say and hear. Words have power. Most people talk in a way that increases body's stress and weakens the immune system and life force (will to live). Sarcasm could literally be killing you. Words can change the way we think and feel. Research has found that speaking and thinking correct thoughts actually changes a person's DNA!

Shut off the TV and NEWS!!! That's a serious form of toxicity that enters through our eyes and brain. Exposure to negative, ugly, disturbing images, sounds, and ideas causes the body to weaken. Get rid of ANYTHING in your life that's toxic - this includes negative people, thoughts, lifestyle things, images, past issues, conscience issues - do some serious soul spring cleaning! Distance yourself from anything that brings you down or doesn't support your well-being.

A German doctor, Dr. Coldwell, has cured more people of cancer than any person in German history without drugs or surgery using stress reduction techniques and correcting people's thoughts.

STRESS
THE BIGGEST KILLER OF ALL

Stress is behind almost every illness known. It literally eats you up. Just ask yourself: what is eating you up? What feelings are you hiding or holding back that are so acidic to your being that they are literally eating holes in you? You can't hold this in or it will kill you. Deal with it or simply walk away and let it go. You need to free yourself of that corrosive issue or relationship. If you hold your feelings in, not letting them out, they fester and that energy has to go somewhere, so it manifests in your body somewhere, eating it up. YOU MUST REDUCE STRESS - it affects every cell in the body. The mind can strengthen or weaken the body in a matter of seconds.

Whatever we think about, we attract. Stop dwelling on the bad stuff and the "what ifs and the unknowns... and focus on what you DO KNOW. Stop attracting the bad stuff with your worrying about it.

LAUGH for no reason - go a little loony - it sends happy vibes to your cells and starts a healing process.

SMILE - something magical happens when you smile at people. You can feel the energy change instantly. It's so overwhelming, many break into tears because of the release.

Don't let the bad stuff get to you. It's part of life. The Universe cannot exist without balance. For every day there is night. But then there will be day again. Be patient and enjoy the ride.
The past is history and what you fear might happen in the future MIGHT NOT! So stop wasting energy and deal with and appreciate what is right in front of you this moment, right now! Start by making others happy. Go out of your way and your healing will start. Always be honest with

yourself and others. Don't play mind games. To be happy, we have to accept what is, and simply deal with it in a calm way, knowing we are free inside.

Look at the people who never get sick. They are always optimistic, easy going, don't let things get to them, don't worry about much, and see the good in things.

A man's life is what his thoughts make of it. "
Marcus Aurelius

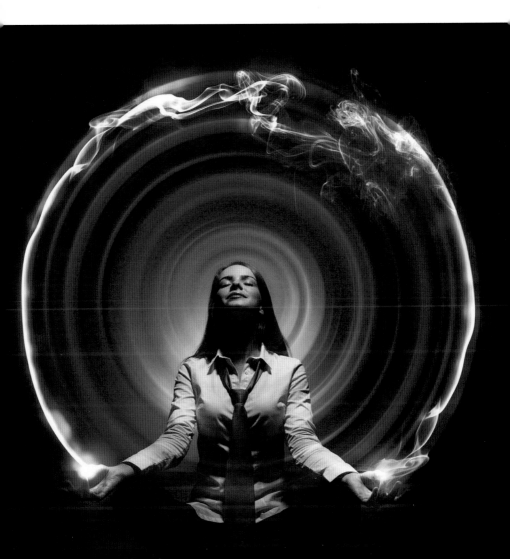

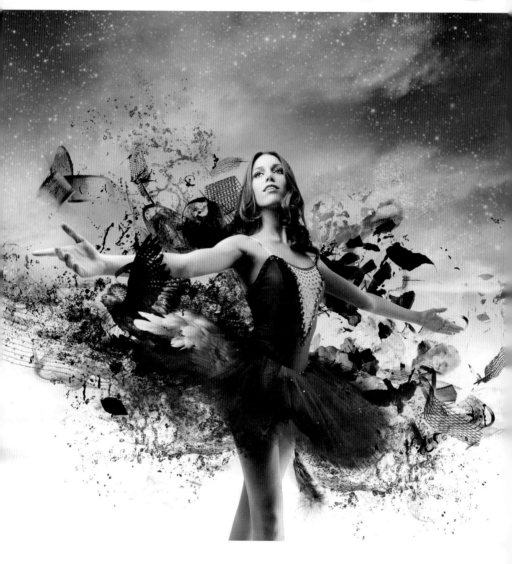

FREE TO BE YOU

If you don't have this, no healthy food in the world is going to save you. I can't stress this enough. If you are not allowed to be YOU, then what you are will die. You are here to be you, not someone else. Your job is to be you. Your mission here on Earth is to offer the world your unique gifts, viewpoints, abilities and style. No one else can be you.

The reason a vast majority of people are unhappy and dying is because they don't think they are free to do what they are here to do. They feel suffocated and held back. This is literally killing them. They spend all their time and energy trying to "fit in" and be like those around them, because they want to be accepted. They are afraid to live.

Everyone is unique, and what we each have to offer is unique. No one else in the world has to offer what we do, in the way we do it. We are a unique piece of a grand glorious puzzle, and if we don't "shape up" to be truly US, then we won't fit into the grand puzzle. Do you see the irony here? We try so hard to "fit in", but that's what's actually stopping us from being what we are designed for- to fit into the space the universe has designed for us. That is the ONLY way we can gain true power, life and freedom. It is our purpose- our reason to live.

Health is just a symptom of how "on track" we are at being ourselves, and doing what we are here to do. The further we are from that design, the less healthy we become. Simply eating the right foods won't give us total health and success. It's a great start, and a very important one, because it helps our machinery run better.

We are a radio antenna. The Universe is constantly sending us messages to follow (guidance) like a cosmic GPS. We can choose to follow it or not. A great number of people don't even hear the message, because there is so much static in their lives. They are so burdened with distractions, commitments, fears, paranoias, health problems, money problems relationship issues and the constant chatter from all the overstimulated lost people and media around them, that they can't possibly hear the message. Their bodies are so clogged from unhealthy crap, it's like a rusted out radio antenna. How can anyone possibly know what their mission is, or even know what their next step is, ...if they can't hear the signal from above? (or deep inside, same thing)

The first step is to UNCLUTTER your life. Get rid of EVERYTHING that's burdening you down. Start right now by getting rid of 20 percent of everything you own. I'm not kidding. Do it right now. That's just a start. Then get away from all the negative people in your life. I don't care if it's your boss, your husband, wife, "friend", neighbor, just do it. I know your saying "yeah sure, easier said than done". At first it will be awkward and difficult, but once you start moving, it becomes easier and easier. I know what else you're thinking- you are afraid you will lose your job, your relationship, your income, a roof over your head,...in other words, your security. This is a major lesson in life that everyone has to learn at some point, better now than later. This lesson is one of the most important lessons you will ever learn. It is so important, I wrote a book about it called "The Prosperity Secret" and it will change your life forever. You can learn more about it and see a video also at HealAnything.com

Let me tell you this. I lived and worked in Hollywood. I had "the" house, "the" car, "the" wife, the nice everything... but I wasn't happy. I had a lot of stuff, but didn't feel fulfilled. I was also dying. Literally. I was bleeding when I went to the bathroom, I had glasses thicker than my finger, I couldn't breathe because I was choking on mucus, and yet I never in my life drank a drop of alcohol, touched a cigarette or even coffee. My relationship was turbulent and neither of us felt fulfilled, no matter how much money we made. It got so bad, one day I just gave up. Literally. I set her free, sold the house, gave everything away and walked into the desert naked, not even knowing if I was going to ever return alive. I didn't care. I gave up.

It was the best thing I ever did.

I owned nothing. I had no identity. I was completely off the map. No more responsibility. I didn't have to answer to anyone. I didn't have to explain myself, pay any bills, meet anyone at a certain time, or do anything. I was free. Wow. I was free. The days, months and years could go by and it wouldn't matter. No more time clock. No agenda.

I woke up lying naked on a rock to behold a beautiful eagle soaring gracefully high overhead in the crystal blue sky. Around me little rabbits, squirrels and lizards quietly hung out nibbling on plants. They were so peaceful. What I learned from them changed my life. It touched me on such a deep level, I saw a new way of living. A new way of looking at life.

There is nothing wrong with having "stuff", or having fun. There is nothing wrong with having a nice house or a fancy car. We just need to learn this stuff is all just on loan to us. We don't own it. It's just a scene in a movie, that's all. If it gets taken away, or falls apart or stolen or burns down, it shouldn't matter. There are many more experiences out there to have. Come on people- LIVE !!!

But this is important, and you must learn this for it to work. Those things must COME TO YOU... you cannot go after them. How? In a nutshell, you must be YOU. This is all explained in the book "The Prosperity Secret". Life will test you. It will challenge and bluff you like a good card game. Remember- it's not the cards you are dealt that matter, but how you play them. Sure you may lose everything. So what. Maybe that stuff wasn't really you anyway. Let go. Losing everything could be the most freeing thing that ever happened to you. I didn't even wait- I just gave it all away. Once you realize you can never starve (weeds are edible remember?), then you start to feel invincible. You can never have "nothing". You are smack in the middle of everything and the entire Universe is around you waiting for you. I was naked in the desert with nothing and within 90 days I was driving a Ferrari. If I can do it, so can you. Do not be afraid to let go of everything burdening you and holding you back. The further the arrow is pulled back, the further it flies once it's let go. Do you want true health? Let go. Now.

THE POWER OF TOUCH

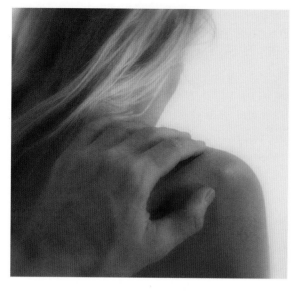

Everything in the Universe is energy. We are electrical beings. Our bodies - nerves, brain, thoughts, heart and so on - run on electricity. When a human being touches the skin of another human being, there is a transfer of energy on many levels. Usually the effect is a good one and we can feel ourselves being charged like a battery, just from that short touch. Soft caressing is super powerful. It can make our whole body quiver with electrical waves. Touch is so vital, so very important.

Animals in tests that had no physical contact with others became ill and died much sooner than those who had physical contact. Want some serious healing energy? Hold someone's hands and look into each others eyes for five or ten minutes. I'll bet it will be so powerfully overwhelming you won't be able to go the whole time - for many it's just too much energy to handle. Try it and hold on as long as you can.

When we lovingly touch anything in life - another person, an animal, plant or even an object - we can feel a healing taking place. No words are needed, yet there is definitely a communication happening... a giving and receiving of love. It changes the very DNA of our cells, and can turn around the very direction of our lives.

HUG PEOPLE!

The Power that Moves the World:
MAKE LOVE for Health

This is one of the most powerful healing forces given to every living thing on the planet. It is a true gift from God. It's pure magic. It's not something to be rushed or taken for granted. Those who worry a lot and have problems being in the moment are sorely missing the tremendous healing benefits this astronomical energy force can bestow. This is validated by numerous studies showing that those who make love all the time live considerably longer than those who don't. Four times a week strengthens our immune system 35% and can cut heart attack, stroke and prostate cancer risk IN HALF! It releases hormones that actually make us younger. The endorphins help us sleep better, and the oxytocin alleviates pain (arthritis, menstrual etc). Menstrual cycles become more regular. It improves

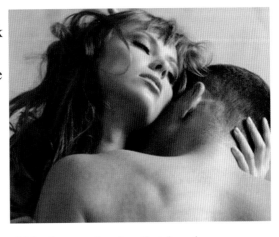

flexibility, firms your butt and abs, and it's the magic glue that bonds couples closer energetically and keeps the relationship strong.

Of course this is if both people are genuinely into it, and into each other, and in love. It shouldn't be selfish, rushed or done out of obligation. There is NO EXCUSE for not making time to make love. Be as spontaneous as you can; if you feel it, show it. It doesn't have to be hot and heavy with orgasms all the time - just a playful and loving show of deep appreciation and affection for the other person. It's not about "getting off", unless both people want that. It's a beautiful energy exchange where both people spontaneously agree without a word spoken to forget the world for a moment and totally let go to the thrill of love and passion. There is nothing like being wanted. To have someone want us so bad, they can't think of anything but becoming one with us - to offer their body completely to us, naked with nothing to hide. The act of submission is deeply touching. They are giving us their only real worldly possession. What an honor that is! When two people bond on such a level, they create more love each time. That's why it's called "Making Love".

"Love is the river of life in the world."

Henry Ward Beecher

This is such an important subject, I plan on writing an entire book on it. An astounding number of people have no idea what magnificence is within their grasp. Many go through their entire life never knowing what is possible, and they die sad, lonely and unfulfilled. What a tremendous waste it is to be given a human body and never fully realize its full potential.

I would like to try and clear some things up. Sex is not dirty. Sensuality is one of the most divine beautiful energies possible on planet Earth. It is so valued, wars have been fought over it and entire civilizations have risen and crumbled from not appreciating or properly understanding it.

When you become enlightened, you realize that there is sensuality in everything. It's a form of true appreciation in seeing beauty in everything, everywhere. It's about being so full of life, you are turned on with every thought, every action in every moment. The very sound of someone's voice becomes healing, and a touch becomes an orgasm.

We have this incredibly powerful force inside us for a reason. There are those who think it's misguided energy and needs to be transmuted into something else whenever we feel it. No! Men who don't ejaculate regularly have double the risk of prostate cancer. Women, breast cancer. Some people think they will become depleted if they do it too much. Only if you do it for the wrong reasons, because that's disrespecting your life-force. But doing it for the RIGHT reasons empowers us to greater heights of being. This is the embodiment of God's celebration of life and love, and those who hold it back become stifled in life, health, finances and happiness. Energy is meant to flow. The more we give, the more we get. USE IT OR LOSE IT. It's a muscle that needs to be worked out. Men who don't ejaculate regularly lose their prostates to cancer. Women's reproductive organs wither and rot if not used. Hormones are what keep us young, healthy, happy and our skin youthful. Sexual energy is not a mistake and it doesn't need to be "channeled" somewhere else and transmuted. We don't take one of God's greatest gifts and try to trade it in for something else. What an insult.

God doesn't make mistakes.

Sexual energy is a gift from God.

It's used to celebrate life. It's not just for creating babies, it's pure Life Force - the power to create anything. It has tremendous power to heal because it creates life. Used correctly, it inspires us to new heights to create amazing things never before dreamt of. It shatters our inner blockages and lets God's energy flow through us like a huge waterfall.

Used incorrectly, it makes our lives empty and meaningless.

Nothing makes the great creator more sad than to see his greatest gift be so disrespected by those who don't fully grasp that what they've been given is in reality a hotline to God and creation itself. When two people love each other so much that they surrender themselves completely and exclusively to each other, and melt their souls and bodies into one, they actually cease to exist as individuals with egos for a short time... and during this glorious moment of letting go ("orgasm" means "little death"), they literally "make love" - all it takes is a flash, a glorious lightning bolt of pure love, and in that miraculous moment we get a pure taste of God - blinding white light surging through our bodies, HEALING EVERYTHING IT TOUCHES: total, pure divine healing energy. And since both bodies are joined, they are melted together energetically, even after they separate. The more "in the moment" the two people are, the more healing the effect is, and the longer it lasts. If you want true healing power, let yourself fall madly in love and celebrate every moment with that person to its absolute fullest. Lose your mind. Excuse my French, but fuck the rest of the world. All that matters is what you have in your arms right here, right now. Do not be a slave to a clock or money or routine. This world and all its responsibilities are temporary. The love you share is forever. God is watching. Celebrate each other completely and fully. Start healing now!!!

"I never knew how to worship until I knew how to love."

Henry Ward Beecher

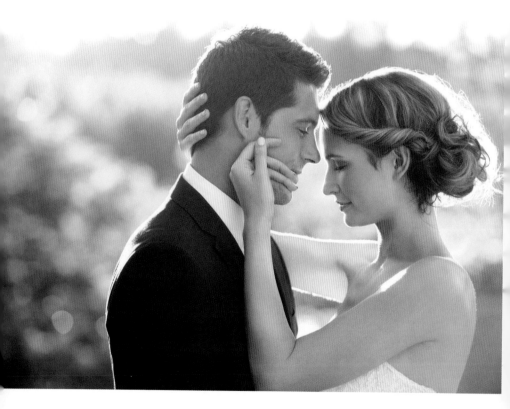

ALONE TIME AND PLACE

It's important to have a loving supportive partner, but it's also equally important to have a bit of "alone" time every day at some point, where we are totally alone ...where nobody can hear us or see us. A place where we can hear our own thoughts and take stock of our lives. Somewhere quiet where we can be undisturbed and reflect on life. It's a time and place to ground out. It could be when everyone leaves the house. It could be when we are in the car alone. It could be sitting in the park watching people... or if we're lucky, a beach somewhere. Sometimes all we have is being in the bathroom alone. Or while we are in the shower. This is medicine for the soul. It calms our stressed-out inner voice by letting it finally be the only one to speak.

Many times stress comes from not being able to hear or speak our inner voice and feelings. Sometimes life is so crazy and distracting with so many people that we have no idea how we personally feel about something, and our inner voice starts to get frustrated. It wants to be heard and paid attention to. We can't force others to do that, but at least we can give it our own personal attention. A quiet place. Just you and your inner voice. Like that faithful loving pet that's waited all day for you to give it some attention. Our inner being needs to be acknowledged, stroked and comforted. It is part of being whole and being healed. Do not neglect that part of you.

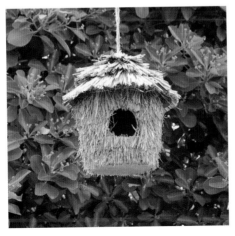

ENERGY WORK
FINDING THE PROPER FREQUENCIES

Everything is just energy. Energy in harmony promotes life, and energy out of sync can be destructive. Listening to soft classical music can soothe and heal, while listening to disturbing sounds can make us ill - like negative news. You know that high pitched squeal truck brakes make? Imagine listening to that sound continuously for a whole hour or two - you know you would not be well at the end of it. The same with nagging partners, friends and family members who complain all the time. You can just feel your energy being sucked. And then there are those beautiful inspirational songs you hear that just pick you up and make you feel invincible. It's all energy. Energy is everything. It heals and destroys. Your job is to align yourself with healing energies. Frequencies that make you feel good. People emit frequencies. Without saying a word, some make you feel good while others drain your energy. Objects, places, sounds, lights and smells can do the same thing. Play music that inspires you and boosts you up. You can tell if it's your frequency or not by how you feel - if it GIVES you energy, that's your vibration... if you feel more tired, drained or irritated by it, it's not you. IMPORTANT: some people have the right frequencies for us but might just be in a bad place right now - don't write them off.
The way you can tell is you feel good being with them on an energetic level, despite the negative things that they say. This is a chance for both of you to heal together. LOVE!

The biggest controllers of your energy vibration are your mind and your heart - use them wisely. What you think and feel sends vibrations to your cells, which heals or destroys. Usually the heart heals and often the mind's overactive paranoia can hurt something beautiful. Don't overthink. Feel. Trust your feelings. Not your thoughts.

Like I said earlier, **healing is not as much about what you take IN, but what you LET GO of and get rid of**. The same goes for energy. Just like bad food that becomes part of our cells and stays stuck in our colon for decades, we accumulate all kinds of old stale crappy energy over the years that we carry with us and we need to get rid of this stuff... like insults that people gave us twenty years ago that still stick with us today: it's eating you up. Get rid of all that stuff!

SCREAM AND SHAKE THERAPY

When you are in that "alone place" that I mentioned earlier, when no one is around... THROW A FIT, scream your freaking head off, jump around, bang the walls, shake like you are being electrocuted, scream as loud as you possibly can. LET IT OUT! You need to clear that bad energy out of your system. Babies and kids intuitively do this and minutes later they are fine. We need to learn from them. Let all that bad energy out. Release it or it will eat you. Once it's out of you, you'll be amazed how fast that space gets filled with healing energy.

Then when in the shower, start singing. This happens intuitively for a reason. We are trying to find our "frequency". Many cultures purposely do chanting. Sing and hold a note, then another, go up and down the scales until you find the note that feels right. Hold it and belt it out loud. Feel it vibrate through your whole body. AAAAAAAH. OOOOOOM. This vibrates all the cells in your body with the healing frequency you need. It helped me when nothing else did. It was my last resort and it worked! If you feel unreleased frustration or pain in your soul, use chanting and screaming. It heals.

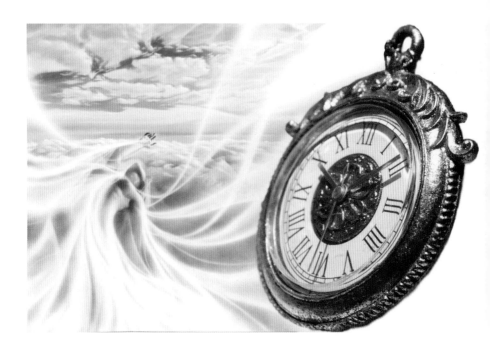

SLEEP

This is the real healing time... and amazingly, you don't have to do anything. Just lay down and close your eyes. How hard is that. This is where the secret magic happens. This is when the night workers put on their hats and fix you... physically, mentally and spiritually. All you have to do is set up the right conditions. Quality sleep is utterly mandatory for true health, longevity, happiness, and well-being.

Next to food, this is one of the most abused and taken-for-granted necessities. If your battery doesn't recharge properly you will wear down, get sick and age. You cannot simply just sleep in late to make up for it. It doesn't work that way. Your body has natural rhythms that are in tune with the Earth, sunlight and so on. If you don't play along, you will not be on the Earth that long. We're supposed to have about eight hours sleep per night. Our body releases healing hormones between 10 pm and 2 am, and we have to be asleep for them to work. Healthy people on average sleep from 10 pm to 6 am.

SPIRITUALITY FAITH and PEACE

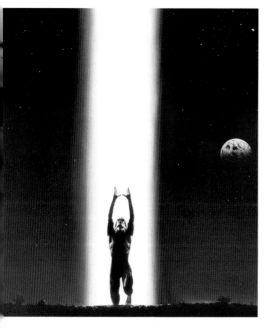

No matter who you are, what race, religion or culture you are from, (even if you are not religious), you know deep inside that you are part of a universal truth that binds and connects everything everywhere. Things may seem random, but you know there are higher levels of consciousness than us. Many times it seems like animals and plants have their acts together better than us humans. We know love is better than hate. We know that courage is better than fear. We cry when someone or an animal makes an unselfish act of love or sacrifice. It gives us hope that there is a level of being better than what we are used to. Countless people have died only to be revived and tell the same amazing stories of what they saw beyond this realm. Every day we experience what can only be described as miracles. Yet every day we are also faced with challenges and tests that question our very faith.

If we knew for sure God existed, we wouldn't be challenged to grow, would we? We'd be spoiled children who take everything for granted. We wouldn't learn and grow because we wouldn't have to. By being tested, we learn about ourselves. The more tests we "pass", the more confidence we gain, and the more we begin to see the infinite intelligence behind this amazing game we are in. This is the school of life and our graduation is eternity. The more we experience and learn, the more peace we feel because we know these are only tests. It's our choice whether or not to pay attention in school and appreciate the teachers, or whether to goof off or be in denial (not pay attention) and have to painfully take the classes over and over again. Have you ever noticed how in school the smart kids were also the most calm, while the party animals seemed to be having all the fun, but if you think about it, deep down inside, they were also the most nervous angst-ridden and needed constant stimulation to keep themselves going and "feeling good". Look how they ended up years later. It's important to have fun, but it should be through genuine appreciation, not artificial stimulation.

When we don't fear reality, we can truly appreciate every little thing in our lives - the sound of a voice, the sparkle in someone's eyes, the soft caress of the wind and the touch of someone's hand. It is when we totally let our guard down and humbly gaze at the world in awe that we start to see the grand design in everything, and how it all speaks the same language. We realize there is a deep current of love connecting everything. We know just like there are unseen radio and satellite waves running through the air, that there are higher frequencies of consciousness and mature understanding out there. Call it whatever you want - God is a good name.

THE QUIET VOICE INSIDE

Close your eyes. Relax. Forget all your worries for a moment. Let go of your thoughts, your fears, your hopes, your incessant mind chatter. Shhh. Listen. There is and has always been a peaceful, quiet voice talking to you. Many times you didn't want to listen because it was telling you to do things that you didn't want to do. It told you to do things that were new, scary or uncomfortable. It asked you to push your comfort level or possibly risk everything you owned. It tested your faith. Many times you knew it was the right thing to do but you still didn't do it. You asked all your friends and family what to do, but didn't trust that voice. Sometimes it was the very last thing you listened to. But no matter what you did, it never abandoned you. Despite what the voice said, you did what you wanted. You just wanted to feel good. The years went by and you got sick, hurt, knocked down, and confused. Yet the voice quietly whispered more suggestions.

172

Why are you fighting the voice? What are you afraid of? Possibly that if you do what it says, life might not be fun anymore? That you may lose everything? What if you did lose everything... and then shortly thereafter got NEW things that were much better than anything you ever had before? The only way to find out is to try. This is called FAITH. You should try it sometime. Do everything that feels right, and nothing that feels wrong, no matter how strong the temptation or fear. This is what every true original religion in the world is simply saying. Don't act from your mind. Act from your HEART. Listen to that quiet voice coming from your heart. Your mind is only a bunch of chatter and crap that people have told you. It will screw you up royally. Your heart on the other hand listens to something much more universal. Animals can't understand words... they never went to school and yet they get along a lot better than we do.

My suggestion is to take a few moments in the day to simply stop... close your eyes and listen. If you are confused, sad, lost or stressed out, then ask for help. Be genuine. Let your guard down. Let the tears come up and out. Cry for help. Let it out. Let it all out.

Be quiet. Listen. Know you are heard. There are forces at work far beyond anything you can comprehend.

Always come from a place of genuineness and love... and because what you put out always comes back, you will get genuineness and love in return. It is the law of the Universe. It might not be in the form you expect, but have patience. You will see and understand why soon enough.

When you send a prayer, always give thanks in advance for what you are about to receive. A genuine "thank you" is usually all the payment required.

Be thankful for everything. Even if you don't understand it yet, be thankful. It is a gift in disguise. Wait and see.

There are only two things: Love and Fear.

Love is the only thing that lasts.

Remember this: Live Fearlessly in Love and watch your entire life change before your eyes!

Start right now.

"Take up one idea. Make that one idea your life
think of it, dream of it, live on that idea.
Let the brain, muscles, nerves, every part of your body,
be full of that idea,
and just leave every other idea alone.
This is the way to success.
That is the way great spiritual
giants are produced."

~ Swami Vivekananda ~

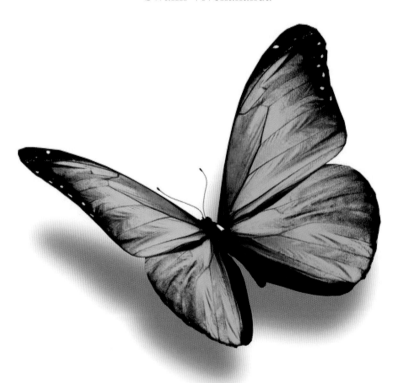

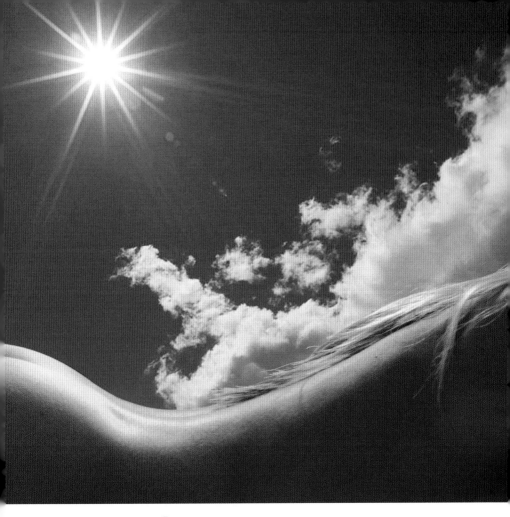

SUNLIGHT
SOLAR ENERGY FOR THE BODY

Let there be light. Sunlight is another heavenly healing gift that has
been misunderstood by modern society. No, it DOESN'T cause cancer.
People who get skin cancer are unhealthy. It's that simple. People in
more primitive countries don't use sunscreen and don't get skin cancer.
Sure many have darker skin, but what happens when you go in the sun?
Your skin gets darker. Protection comes naturally. Dark-skinned people
in the United States are starting to get skin cancer - what's the difference?
Diet and lifestyle! Don't believe anyone who tells you sunshine causes
melanoma. What a crock. Just the opposite. In studies all over the world,

as sun exposure increases, malignant skin cancer risk goes down. In the sunniest parts of Australia, lifeguards have lower skin cancer rates than office workers. That's right: more sun, less cancer. Then how come a number of people get melanoma who go in the sun? Because they are TOXIC. They eat wrong, smoke, drink, and fill their bodies with all kinds of processed chemical crap. Their livers are clogged and not working right anymore and their kidneys are so toxic that the blood has to push the toxins out through the skin, where it gets baked by the sun into the skin cells, causing melanoma.

The same goes for wrinkles. Sugar cross links the proteins in the skin causing skin to lose elasticity and wrinkle. Almost everything in the modern diet has wrinkles. There are blond people from northern Europe who travel the world in sunny tropical places who are super tanned but don't have lots of wrinkles. The difference? They eat healthier. Health comes from inside, not something you slather on from the outside. Sunscreen is one of the most toxic things you can put on your skin! It causes more skin cancer than anything. Look at the label. You are literally basting and baking those chemicals into your skin cells! Want cancer? Slather that crap on.

God doesn't make mistakes. We are designed to be in the sun. People who don't get enough sunlight start having all kinds of physical, mental and emotional problems. Bones go soft (a condition called rickets), depression sets in (the highest suicide rates are in places with the least sunlight), hormone levels and immunity plummets and people become sick.
On the other hand, people who DO get Sun:
-have more energy, feel better, happier
-have stronger immune systems, get sick less
-have denser, stronger bones
-have stronger muscles
-have richer blood
-have healthier nerves
-sunlight increases the amount of iron in their blood (gives tanned look)

176

Consider these facts:
-USA cancer rates are highest in the states with least sunshine
-sunshine may reduce breast cancer by up to 40% and ovarian cancer by 80%
-direct sun exposure kills most forms of mold, fungus and yeast
-sun exposure normalizes hormone levels, raises sex drive and fertility
-Vitamin D, which assists the mineralizing of bones, is formed when skin is exposed to sunlight

I don't put anything on my skin personally, but you can use coconut oil or olive oil. Don't put anything on your skin that you wouldn't eat. Trans-dermal (through the skin) is the fastest way to get a substance into your bloodstream, like the nicotine patch. Stay away from poisonous sunscreen! You NEED sunlight to be healthy, but you need to be healthy to get a lot of sun. My suggestion is to put some jojoba oil on your skin & get 20 minutes of sun exposure a day (while eating right and detoxing).

NATURE'S SUNSCREEN

The grand design of nature is amazing. Again, primitive people and animals don't use sunscreen and don't get skin cancer. What's the secret? They get their "sunscreen" from what they EAT. And what might that be you may ask? Drum roll please... GREEN leafy foods. These contain chlorophyll. Why do you think plants, with their delicate leaves, don't fry and wither in the sun? Chlorophyll. That green magic property that protects plants is the same stuff that protects us, once we consume it. Aloe Vera is edible sunscreen that protects you from the inside when you eat it. It grows in the desert for a reason!

Without sunlight, the bones cannot become calcified. Sunlight builds the immune system and increases oxygenation of the skin. It lowers blood sugar. Sunlight brings more blood to the skin surface, which helps heal cuts, bruises and rashes. Open wounds and broken bones heal faster in sunlight. Sunlight improves eyesight and hormones. Get at least thirty minutes of sunlight each day. There is no mistake in nature. We need sunlight. Plants do it. Animals do it. You do it!

SUMMARY

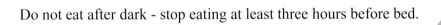

Cooking is a big waste of time.

Fast one day a week.

Rest one day a week - no work.

Do not eat after dark - stop eating at least three hours before bed.

If you have a disease, you are unclean inside body, mind and spirit

Cleanse as much as possible, especially the INSIDE of your body and mind.

No bread, cereal, coffee, smoke, alcohol, meat, dairy, sugar, salt, or cooked food.

Let go of everything in your life that's negative or burdening you.

Have metal tooth fillings removed.

Less sweet stuff and more greens. Include more bitter stuff

Try to stay away from things that grow under the ground: carrots, beets, potatoes, BUT eat the green leaves on top, especially carrot and beet greens, but potato and tomato greens are toxic, don't touch them

The only thing shown to conclusively lengthen lives is NOT eating very much. The people who eat the least live the longest.

Grow and make your own food as much as possible - even raw food places try to save money. They give you one scoop of something where you would use five at home.

Reduce STRESS. It's involved in almost all illness.

Sunbathe naked daily for twenty minutes.

Laugh, smile, hug, love, dance, sing.

Give stuff away: lighten your load.

Eat to Live instead of living to eat.

Be more thankful.

Be honest.

Be good to others.

Get massages. Treat yourself well.

Good thoughts = health, bad thoughts = disease.

Write down your goals so that they become more focussed and real.

Read "The Prosperity Secret" over and over regularly

Read "Instructions for a New Life" over and over regularly

Walk barefoot on natural ground (grass, stone, sand, earth).

If you are depressed or confused, CLEANSE: do an enema or fast.

Bed: 10pm - 6am. Try 9 pm- 5 am

What the caterpillar calls the end of the world,
the master calls the butterfly."

Richard Bach

IF IT ISN'T WORKING:

1 - You aren't doing enough and your doses are too low

-more enemas ****
-more green juices
-more exercise
-more sleep
-more happiness

2 - You are still doing something that's bad for you

-you are still eating sweet stuff and cooked food (cooking breaks down fiber into simple sugars). Stop the fruit juice!
-still sneaking bread in?
-stress: the number one source - check relationships, job, money, bills, responsibilities. Get off the internet
-do you still have metal tooth fillings?
-are you taking ANY kind of medication?
-check if anything has wheat, sugar, milk, cheese, preservatives.
-alcohol
-inhaling cigarette smoke (one night of second hand smoke in a club is equivalent to 2 packs!)
-are you taking mainstream supplements? (you won't believe what some of these are made from)
- carbonated drinks (even water)? Carbonation shuts down calcium absorption for twelve hours.
-the flour in those "healthy wraps" has wheat, gluten and trans-fats. Same goes for tortillas, tacos, burritos etc.
-no white rice
-no cereal
-less dehydrated food - cookies, crackers, granola, dried fruit etc.
-are you sneaking a chocolate cookie when no one's looking? No baked goods or sugar!

-are you sitting all day, not enough exercise?
-check your dressings for dairy & bad oils like canola, safflower, soy, peanut, vegetable.
-no soy milk, soy cheese, meat substitutes etc.
-too many nuts? Are they soaked first?
-check your stomach acid level (does beet juice stain your poop or pee)?
-check your water. Plastic? flouride? chlorine? Rusty metal pipes?
-chemical fumes from computers, cars, carpeting, plastics, workplace.
-what are you using for laundry detergent, shampoo, conditioner, soap?
-gas furnace, stove, gas heating
-carpeting; new carpeting is toxic (synthetic fumes), and old carpeting is full of mold, fungus, mites, parasites, and more disgusting things than you can imagine. The padding is a major source of toxic fumes.
-no TV or news.
-do you really want to get better? I'm not kidding. Some people love the attention and pity. They want to be martyrs ("I would die for you"). Usually people who feel they aren't getting enough attention in a relationship do this. It's their way of trying to get more love. Is this you? Many people aren't even aware they are doing this. They actually WANT to be sick, because they want to be loved more and nursed by their spouse or family. The motive isn't a bad one and the wrong thing is to be angry at people like this. They need love and understanding. Just know that wanting to be ill for attention actually drives people away. It backfires. Nobody wants to be around negative, pitiful people.

The mind is very powerful and can sabotage anything. Ask yourself seriously: "How am I benefiting from not being healthy?". Think about this for a moment. What are you getting out of it? Empathy from friends? More attention from your loved ones? (Poor them)... or... do you want to even be alive anymore? Have you lost your will? Have you done what you came here to do and your work is done? Moving on is not necessarily a bad thing. Just know that you don't have to do it in a painful, dramatic way that could possibly hurt others. Be loving in everything you do. You are in control. Nobody controls you unless you let them. Be free. Be you. Live life your way.

Life does not have to be painful near the end. Pure raw foodists who are happy with their lives are healthy and full of life until the very end. When their time has come, they become incredibly peaceful, as their body fades away within a matter of days. As this happens, their essence distances itself from the body (an out of body experience), so that no pain is felt. It is actually a beautiful transcending experience for those in the right space, without fear and filled with nothing but love.

THE BIGGEST HEALER OF ALL:

Love

"Love is the beauty of the soul."

St. Augustine

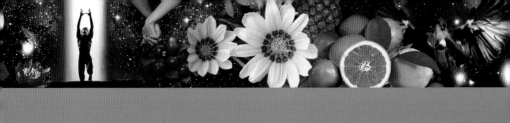

FINAL WORD

Take a good look at yourself. If your body is sick, it means your mind or spirit is sick. Your spirit is what keeps your body alive. Do whatever it takes to nourish your spirit and soul. Don't wait for others to do it for you. You are in charge of your life, no one else.

This is not just a matter of taking herbs or drugs to hide symptoms - the issues that cause this sickness must be addressed. You MUST stop what's causing the problem in the first place! Eating bread, sugar, milk and animal products docs not just give us pimples, it throws our whole body off balance, which throws off our way of thinking and the energy we convey to others. The energy we create attracts or pushes away success, prosperity, health, relationships, longevity, etc. Energy affects everything. That's why we are attracted to healthy, successful people and avoid unhealthy, unsuccessful people. Sadness can literally make us ill and cause disease. Health is what we put into our bodies, mind and spirits. It is the result of what we eat, drink, watch, read, say, think and do. Our parents gave us a vehicle in which to live. What we do with it is our choice.

This will be your great test. This is your gauntlet. Make it through the cleansing and every other problem in your life that you will ever face will be easy after that. This doesn't just cleanse your body, but your mind and soul too, because it is a test of character and it builds strength. You will be rewarded in more ways than you can imagine, because your mind, body and soul will clear up so much that you will be able to take on the world. You will be rewarded with a new body. You will look in the mirror and go "WOW - WHO IS THAT?" You will get a hormone rush just looking at yourself. Other people will too, when they look at you. Like a cadet at the military academy, you will have earned your stripes.

Not everybody has the strength to do this. They want to go back to their comfort foods, and age and get sick and die young. Don't let that be you. A few donuts aren't worth dying for. Many of you will say: "yeah, but those few donuts aren't going to kill me. Or that one pizza. Or that one soft drink." True. But the odds are that you'll have another one a few days later. Or a week later. Then another. That's like putting a bit of sand or water in your car's gas tank every day, or week. Pretty soon you have a clogged up, rusted out car that one day just won't work any more. Don't let that be you!

This book should give you the info you need to dramatically change your life. I know to many of you, this is new territory and might seems a bit scary and strange, especially after a lifetime of misinformation and bad habits passed on to you from parents, friends and society. It's really pretty simple, but our minds are afraid of new things and unfamiliar territory. They try to protect us from what they don't know. The irony is, this has been HURTING us, because our minds have been told all kinds of garbage, and that's why people are so sick, tired, run down, depressed, unhappy, unsuccessful, irritated and confused.

I get lots of emails every day from all over the world (about 300), and I just don't have time to answer them... especially when they start asking health questions. I can't "fix" you with one quick email, because there are so many factors to consider-. There is no "magic pill". That's why I wrote

184

this book. You need to take a good look at your life and what habits made you what you are, and if you want to change, you have to change your habits. Be sure to check out MarkusFAQ.com for answers to frequently asked questions. You need to start taking control of yourself. That's what I'm about- giving you the inspiration and strength to not need anything or anyone outside of yourself anymore. This is true self-empowerment.

The answers are usually simpler than you think. We were born with everything we need. Nature is perfect. All you need to do is understand it a bit better. And when you do, you will be in love with life and amazed at how awesome and miraculous it is. There is pure genius in the grand design of life and how it all connects. If bugs can understand it, so can you. Your overly paranoid, analytical, fearful mind just got in the way. Let me help clear it out and get you on the path of true life again. Get younger. Never get sick again!

Be alive. Be sexy. Never get sick again. Be the envy of your friends. Show them this works and maybe they'll do it too. This is how the world will change. It starts here and now with you.

The cure for everything is: Truth - Nature - Love.

When you are one with nature, she is one with you.

Love and Light,

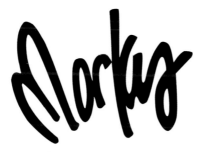

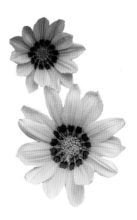

Send me your testimonials! Email me at **Markus@BeautifyLife.com**
If you have shipping questions- email **Info@MarkusProducts.com**
* *Remember I cannot answer health questions*

OTHER MARKUS PRODUCTS

You can get everything at **HealAnything.com**

FREE FOOD AND MEDICINE WORLDWIDE EDIBLE PLANT BOOK

The definitive book on edible plants found all over the world. Over 2,500 beautiful full color images covering over 1,000 plants and what health conditions they have been historically used for. What common neighborhood plants make a great shampoo, soap and toothpaste? What flowers and common house plants are edible? 480 pages of fascinating facts and beautiful images. It teaches plant basics, and how you can grow your own and what plants are toxic.This is as packed as it gets. Those wild plants growing just outside your house are some of the best free food and medicine you could ever have! A 2 lb field guide. **EdiblePlantGuide.com**

FREE FOOD AND MEDICINE 5 DVD Set Documentary

A fascinating, highly informative journey showing how those wild plants growing outside your door have been used for thousands of years as FREE FOOD and MEDICINE. All plants have a purpose. Get to know your local wild plants and what they are good for. People all over the world are rediscovering these magical gifts of nature. Set includes a free wild foods recipe booklet. This set shows the most common plants found worldwide. See the video trailer and buy the set at **FreeFoodandMedicine.com**

LOVE ON A PLATE, the Uncookbook- Your idea of healthy food

is about to change forever. You can still eat pizza, pasta, bacon, cheese, pop tarts, Kung Pao unchicken, Pasta Pomodoro and all the pies, cookies and cakes you want without sacrificing your health. In fact, as sinful as this food seems, it might actually make you feel better than you've ever felt in your life. This is an amazing breakthrough in health food - all made without meat, dairy, wheat, sugar or anything unnatural. Yet it looks and tastes like the real thing. Everything is simple and easy. The beautiful pictures alone make this a collectors coffee table book. Give this work of love to as many friends as you can! 232 page hardcover. Yes this is what Markus and Cara eat! See the video at **HealthyCookbook.com**

The PROSPERITY SECRET hardcover book and DVD set
Successful people know that prosperity has nothing to do with money
(that's just a side effect). It comes from having the courage to lose
everything and follow your dream to help others in a way that's
meaningful to them. Success has nothing to do with talent, hard work, who
you know, or luck. This book is not new age esoteric fluff. Forget power
of attraction- this is solid simple truth and it works. This will change your
life forever. See **ProsperitySecret.com**

HEAL YOUR FACE by Healing your Body - softcover book
Unhappy with your face? Your body is trying to tell you something.
Every line, wrinkle, spot, mole and crease means something. They did
NOT just randomly show up on your face. Every part of your face is
connected to an organ or body part. If that body part is not functioning
properly, this will show up on your face. No amount of cream will change
that. If you want to improve your face, you must improve your health.
And lucky for you, your face tells you exactly what's wrong with you.
Forget plastic surgery - you can do it yourself. After reading this book,
you will never look at people the same way again. You will instantly be
able to tell what issues they (or you) have. And they will wonder why you
now look twenty years younger! **HealFace.com**

RAW VEGAN MUSCLE 3 Disc Set - how to get muscles without
eating meat or dairy. Featuring raw vegan professional bodybuilders, and
even a Las Vegas cab driver who eats for only six dollars a day and yet has
huge muscles. These people eat half what they used to, only work out two
or three times a week and yet look like supermen. Be inspired and learn
their secrets. See the video trailer at: **HealthyMuscleDVD.com**

INSTRUCTIONS FOR A NEW LIFE - The pocketbook that will
change your life. Your intuitions have been right. It's time you started
following them. No more wromg relationships wrong jobs and destructive
habits just to make it another few hours. Start Living. Now. It's easier than
you think. No more confusion, desperation, pain and emptiness.
See **NewLifeBook.com**

MY READY-TO-GO HERBAL FORMULAS

You can mix your own herbs and formulas (sources are listed on following pages) or simply buy my ready-to-go formulas at **MarkusProducts.com** Keep checking for new stuff. I aim to put out only the very best, most affordable and useful healing products possible.

DAILY WILD GREENS POWDER- Energy, vitamins and minerals for busy people on the go who don't have wild greens growing nearby, or don't have the time, simply put a couple spoonfuls of this amazing powder in a glass of morning water or smoothie. One of the most nutrient-dense powders you can get. Feel the power of WILD greens! Great for traveling and work. See **MarkusGreens.com** or **WildForce.com**

SUPER PLANT PROTEIN-Made from the best raw vegan protein on Earth! Competitors' products don't even come close to matching its quality and rare ingredients, like durian, prickly pear and pine nuts, one of the highest sources of protein of any nut or seed, but too expensive for others to use. Try it for a month and watch the results in the mirror!
See **MarkusProtein.com** or **WildForce.com**

PARASITE-FREE - one of the most powerful and effective parasite formulas on the market - 100% natural herbal formula. Everyone has parasites. They are the silent cause of many illnesses. Watch the scary video at **ParasiteFree.net**

AGE-FREE - powerful antioxidant protection product against AGING and free radical damage. Contains many of the most potent adaptogens that benefit ageless skin, heart, circulation, arteries, keep hair from graying, provide better vision, blood pressure, lower cholesterol, fight infection, promote liver cell regeneration and even rebuild dendrite growth in the brain! Ingredients & benefits listed on website. **AgeFreeFormula.com**

FREE-LIVER - your liver is your body's filter. It's your most important organ. All illness starts with a clogged liver. If you are tired a lot, you need to clean out your liver! Contains Chanca Piedra - an herb that helps dissolve kidney and gall stones. Recommended! **MarkusLiverFormula.com** Be sure to see the Liver video to learn all about this important organ.

CHARCONITE - a super powerful combination of activated charcoal and bentonite to absorb ANYTHING toxic inside you, plus some herbs to help push it through your digestive system. Perfect for managing gas, food poisoning, toxic environmental poisons, bad food and even toxins created by illnesses and parasites. It goes through your system absorbing anything bad. See the video at **Charconite.com**

FREE-COLON - cleaning out the colon is the FIRST thing you should do before anything else. This formula helps get things moving without giving you the runs. It works awesomely ! See video at **FreeColon.com**

NIGHT REBUILD - For people under a lot of stress & those entering middle age. Night time is when hormones are produced & the body heals itself, but you must be asleep for this to happen.This formula helps promote restful sleep and hormone production. Other than the wild greens, this is the most important formula for people in the modern world. This is exactly the formula Cara and I personally use, and in my mid 50's, I have the hormones of a teenager. Say goodbye to night sweats and hello to great SLEEP. If you are serious about regenerating health, youth and vitality, this is your formula! See video at **NightFormula.com**

SUPER HERBAL VITAMIN C- There is no natural herbal vitamin C anywhere that even comes close to the power of these plant sources. Vitamin C helps convert cholesterol to adrenal hormones. Lack of vitamin C is one of the biggest reasons for collagen loss leading to wrinkles, aging, weakened arteries, and immune deficiency. Stress and stimulants like caffeine cause vitamin C deficiencies, so people in the modern world NEED vitamin C! Take as much of this stuff as you want. **MarkusVitaminC.com**

Energy Formula- Most energy formulas cheat by blasting you with sugar or overstimulating your system with fast-energy substances and herbs that jolt the system just so you can make it another few hours. This overstimulation ultimately burns out your adrenals in the long run, leaving you even more burned out than before, with low hormones and accelerated aging. This formula is designed to rebuild adrenals and work on a much deeper level with longer-lasting results. See **MarkusEnergy.com**

TRIM FORCE- This amazing formula does multiple things. It burns fat you already have and turns it into energy, and it stops new sugar and starches you eat from absorbing into the body, thus helping prevent new fat from forming. Even more amazing, is that - in the powder form - it even helps block your ability to taste sugar and making sugar taste funky, thus reducing the desire for it. See **TrimForce.com**

SEA MOSS- Seaweeds are really high in minerals, protein, iodine and this one in particular helps plump up your skin and food. This is the real stuff, and it's good for you. (Watch the video!) Don't use Irish Moss powder or flakes because it's been cooked dry in an oven and doesn't have the great qualities anymore that this fresh stuff does. Not only can you make beautiful desserts with this, but your skin, hair and thyroid will thank you. See **SeaMoss101.com**

MarkusSweet- All natural zero calorie sweetener, zero insulin response

Prebiotic Fiber Blend- Food for your gut flora probiotics to thrive

FREE LIVING 101 6 disk set
Everything you need to live is within one mile of where you live. Garry Tibbo is living proof of this. He lives in a normal suburban home but doesn't need a grocery store or even a job. He eats wild plants and makes money recycling. This is NOT a poverty lifestyle. It healed his serious health conditions. Gary saved enough money to buy over seven hundred acres of forest and farm land in the country! He lives in Toronto Canada, where it snows in the winter. If he can do this, so can you. Forget the economy. This is a new way of living. Free Living.
See the video trailer at **FreeLiving101.com**

DreamChaser- The inspiring true story of how Markus went from being a sickly little boy that was beat up at school and lost everything multiple times over in life to making his own 2.5 million dollar fantasy motion picture that inspired people all over the world. Lots of illustrations, sketches and behind-the-scene color images explaining how Markus did the impossible. See the inspiring video at **Dreamchaserbook.com**

MARKUS PAINTINGS, The Collectors Coffee table Book

We need to take time to enjoy the beauty this world has to offer. Whenever you need to escape the stress of daily life, pick up this book and escape into some of the images- they will take you to another reality of peace, beauty and overwhelming calmness. Looking at this book is a Zen experience. You can feel yourself being pulled into the landscapes, and almost immediately feel yourself being inspired with creative energy and revived spirit.
MarkusPaintingsBook.com

TO THE ENDS OF TIME- the Movie- This is the epic movie Markus made in 1994 for 2.5 Million that played in theaters all over the world. It's a romantic storybook fantasy with flying ships, castles above the clouds and a love story that transcends time. A film for the whole family starring Christine Taylor, Sarah Douglas, Tom Schultz and Joss Ackland. Newly remastered 92 min DVD.

EBOOKS ON ANY HEALTH CONDITION- instantly download over 70 downloadable eBooks on any health condition, everything from Alzheimers to Zits, from Candida to Prostate and Breast Cancer. These PDFs explain what the symptoms are, what causes them and what to do about it. If you followed everything in this book, chances are you will not have these problems anymore, but the supplemental ebooks also mention specific herbs and remedies that can help different conditions. They will also help you understand why you have a condition, which is probably even more important. There are over 3000 pages of information - a lifetime of research! They are available at: **MarkusEbooks.com**

To get my latest news, updates and videos, go to
MarkusNews.com
simply enter your name and email address.

If you need specific information or want to know more on your condition, I have over 70 downloadable eBooks on everything from Alzheimers to Zits. These PDFs explain what the symptoms are, what causes them and what to do about it. If you followed everything in this book, chances are you will not have these problems anymore, but the supplemental ebooks also mention specific herbs and remedies that can help different conditions. They will also help you understand why you have a condition, which is probably even more important. There are over 3000 pages of information - a lifetime of research! They are available at: **MarkusEbooks.com**

My supplemental PDF booklets mention specific herbs to take for conditions. Be responsible when taking herbs.

HERB AND PLANT SAFETY

Get to know which plants are which. Plants and herbs are powerful, just like medicine. Start with the ones you know and avoid the ones you don't. Study and learn about the rest before taking them. Some plants are poisonous - for example, common oleander - all parts of this plant are poison. Poison Hemlock is poison (not to be confused with a hemlock tree which isn't poisonous. Then there are plants that can do miraculous things, but are harmful if not used correctly - these include poke, belladonna, lobelia, foxglove and jimson weed. That's why I suggest you start by getting the **Free Food and Medicine Worldwide Edible Plant Guide**. Herbs can interact with prescription medicine. They can also interact with other herbs, making them stronger or weaker or prolonging the effect. Pregnant women should be careful. Some herbs are uterine stimulants and could cause abortion... BUT other herbs can counteract that... so know your herbs and consult with a specialist first.

Fruit Trees and plants shipped to you- EdibleLandscaping.com

Where to get Herb Powders (other than mine)
Below are places to get herbs and other healing things...
so you can mix your own concoctions:
HerbalCom.com
(888) 649-3931 (billed as AmeriHerb, Inc.) 515-232-8614
ZNaturalFoods.com
Mountain Rose Herbs MountainRoseHerbs.com 800-879-3337
Wilderness Family Naturals - wildernessfamilynaturals.com 800-945-3801
TheRawFoodWorld.com Matt and Angela Monarch's site
LuckyVitamin - LuckyVitamin.com   888-635-0474
Starwest-Botanicals.com
FrontierCoop.com
LivingEarthHerbs.com
DiscountNaturalHerbs.com
FloridaHerbHouse.com
OsageGardens.com
Remember the Asian markets!

TOCOTRIENOLS (Rice Bran Solubles)- RicePlex.com

Red raspberry seed powder (Ellagitannin, Ellagic acid) available at:
Scientific Medical Devices, Inc.*** smdi.org 770-889-6240

MEYER LEMONS can be grown indoors- FourWindsGrowers.com for
baby meyer lemon trees.

Diatomaceous Earth - EarthWorksHealth.com

HEALTHY PET FOOD
Amorepetfoods.com - best for individual packages
Huntjeni.com
Wildside Salmon Freeze-dried cat treats - catconnection.com

Dehydrator, juicers - healthnutalternatives.com 800-728-1238
TheRawFoodWorld.com (Matt Monarch's company - raw foods,
appliances, books etc)

SEAWEED

TheSeaweedMan.com
Maine Coast Seaweed Co (sun/wind dried) 207-546-2875
Goldminenaturalfood.com 800-475-3663 seaweed, macrobiotic, Nama Shoyu
Country Life Natural Foods - 800-456-7694 clnf.org
Living Tree Community - organic grown foods and UNpressed olive oil
livingtreecommunity.com 800-260-5534

NON-TOXIC DENTISTRY

Holistic non toxic dentistry:
Scientific Health 800-331-2303
Referrals for Huggins dentists.

International Academy of Oral and Toxology 863-420-6373 Metal-free
dentists.

Foundation for toxic-free dentistry - send self-addressed, stamped
envelope to Box 608010, Orlando, Fl 32860

Environmental Dental Association 800-388-8124

American Academy of Biological Dentistry 831-659-5385
831-659-2417

Ashwood Holistic Dentistry, Ventura California 805-654-0880
AshwoodHolisticDentistry.com

RAW FOOD HEALING CENTERS AND RETREATS

Raw food healing places are popping up everywhere- do an internet search
for your area.
Ann Wigmore Institute
Box 429 Rincon, Puerto Rico 00677 USA
787-868-6307 fax 787-868-2430

Ann Wigmore Foundation
P.O. Box 399
San Fidel, NM 87049
info@wigmore.org
Phone 505/5552-0595 Fax 505/552-0595

Hippocrates Health Institute & Spa   Email: hippocrates@worldnet.att.net
1443 Palmdale Court
West Palm Beach, FL 33411
561-471-8876, 800-842-2125 fax: 561-471-9464
Tree of Life Rejuvenation Center
PO Box 1080, Patagonia, AZ 85624
520-394-2520 fax: 520-394-2099
Email: tlrc@dakotacom.net

Optimum Health Institute http://www.optimumhealth.org
San Diego - 6970 Central Avenue, Lemon Grove, CA 91945
(800) 993-4325 or (619) 464-3346
E-mail: optimum@optimumhealth.org

OHI Austin - 265 Cedar Lane, Cedar Creek, TX 78612
(800) 993-4325 or (512) 303-4817
E-mail: reservations.austin@optimumhealth.org

Annapurna Retreat & Spa
538 Adams St.
Port Townsend, WA, 98368
annapurna@olympus.net
Phone 1-800-868-2662 Fax 1-360-379-0711

Healing Waters Health Center
1016 N. Davis Drive
Arlington, Texas 76012
cldarton@aol.com
Phone (817)275-4771

Shinui Living Foods Retreat & Learning Center
1085 Lake Charles Dr.
Roswell, GA 30075
gideongraff@mindspring.com
Phone 770 992-9218

Creative Health Institute
112 West Union City Road
Union City, Michigan 49094
517-278-6260   creativehealth@hotmail.com

FINLAND
The Institute of Living Food on Åland Ltd.
22930 Fiskö
Åland, Finland
phone & fax: +358-28-56 285

ENGLAND
Elaine Bruce - Living Foods Centre
Holmleigh, Gravel Hill Ludlow, SY8 1QS, UK
Phone 00944 (0)1584 875308 Fax 00944 (0)1584 875778

NON TOXIC COSMETICS
REAL PURITY - realpurity.com 800-253-1694
Eccobella.com 877-696-2220 ext 19
Primal Life Organics Beauty Products http://www.primallifeorganics.com
100Percent Pure http://www.100percentpure.com
Jenulence http://www.jenulence.com
Lavera Organic Mascara http://www.lavera.com
Aubrey Organics http://www.aubrey-organics.com
Aveda http://www.aveda.com
Coconut Oil (Used as Makeup Remover and for Dry Elbows, Lips & Feet)
Mychelle http://www.mychelle.com
RealPurity.com "From nature to You" http://www.RealPurity.com
LUSH Fresh Handmade Cosmetics https://www.lush.co.uk note: not all
Lush products are 100% natural, read the ingredients to make sure they are
free of parabens, fragrance, phthalaytes etc

HAIR CARE
Bragg's Organic Apple Cider Vinegar & Olive Oil   bragg.com
Miracle II soap http://www.miraclesoap.com
Beautiful On Raw Products http://www.beautifulonraw.com
Primal Life Organics Beauty Products http://www.primallifeorganics.com
100Percent Pure http://www.100percentpure.com
Morroco Method Int'l http://www.MorroccoMethod.com
Herbal Choice Mari http://www.herbalchoicemari.com Hair repair oil &
skin care products very inexpensive Vegan, Organic
Lovely Lady Products http://www.LovelyLadyProducts
Aubrey Organics http://www.aubrey-organics.com

LUSH Fresh Handmade Cosmetics https://www.lush.co.uk note: not all Lush products are 100% natural, read the ingredients to make sure they are free of parabens, fragrance, phthalaytes etc
Aveda http://www.aveda.com

HAIR COLORING

Logona Naturkosmetik Germany http://www.Logona.com Now in Whole Foods
Color Me Organic http://www.colourmeorganic.com
Herbatint natural colours http://www.herbatintusa.com
Morroco Method Int'l http://www.MorroccoMethod.com
Aveda http://www.aveda.com Company is 100% wind powered, products created at Aveda's botanical laboratory on the 59 acre certified wildlife habitat in Minnesota. Packaging cartons made from 100% recycled materials
NatureTint plant based permanent hair color- no ammonia, no parabens, no resorcinol. has peroxide. http://www.naturtintusa.com
LUSH Hair color bars https://www.lush.co.uk/article/henna-safe-alternative-synthetic-hair-dye

SKIN CLEANSERS (SOAP)

Miracle II http://www.miraclesoap.com Skin moisturizer, neutralizer liquid and Neutralizer gel
Bragg's Organic Apple Cider Vinegar bragg.com
Beautiful On Raw Products http://www.beautifulonraw.com
Dr. Bronner's All purpose Soap https://www.drbronner.com
100Percent Pure http://www.100percentpure.com
Morroco Method Int'l http://www.MorroccoMethod.com
Herbal Choice Mari http://www.herbalchoicemari.com
Lovely Lady Products http://www.LovelyLadyProducts.com
Aubrey Organics http://www.aubrey-organics.com
Herbal Choice Mari http://www.herbalchoicemari.com
Lovely Lady Products http://www.LovelyLadyProducts.com
Aubrey Organics http://www.aubrey-organics.com
Aveda http://www.aveda.com
Nava Naturals http://www.navanaturalskincare.com

LIP CARE

Bee Magic medicinemamasapothecary.com
Egyptian Magic http://www.egyptianmagic.com
Burt's Bees Lip Balm http://www.burtsbees.com
Badger Organic Lip Balm http://www.badgerbalm.com
Herbal Choice Mari http://www.herbalchoicemari.com
Aubrey Organics http://www.aubrey-organics.com
100Percent Pure http://www.100percentpure.com
Aveda http://www.aveda.com
Jenulence http://www.jenulence.com
Mychelle http://www.mychelle.com
Bella Organics http://www.lovebelloaorganics.com

DEODORANT *(If you are really clean you don't need deodorant)*

Miracle II Natural Deodorant http://www.miraclesoap.com
Herbal Choice Mari http://www.herbalchoicemari.com
Aubrey Organics http://www.aubrey-organics.com
RealPurity.com "From nature to You" http://www.RealPurity.com
Bella Organics http://www.lovebelloaorganics.com

But remember...

You don't need to go anywhere or spend lots of money to heal.

**The best healing center is inside you right now,
in your own home.**

Stop depending on things and people outside of yourself.

You were born with everything you need.

Heal Yourself

Right Now !

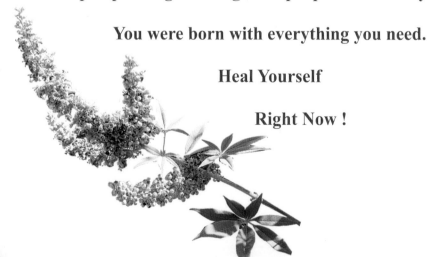

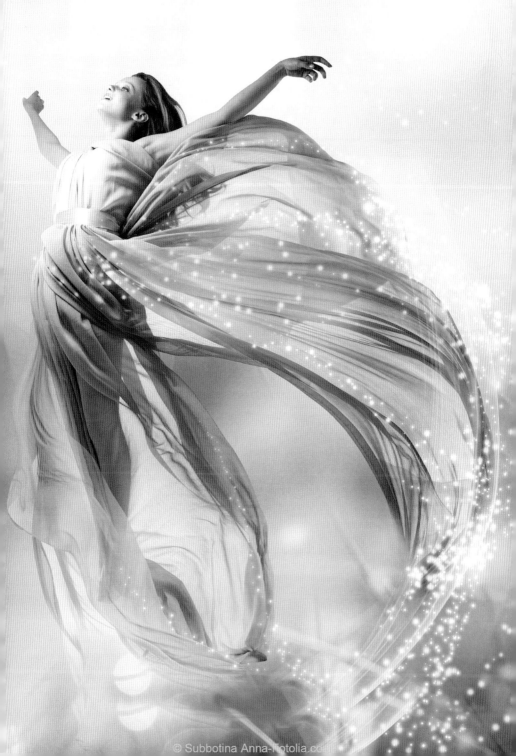

Your Time has Come

In my 50's, I am actually younger than when I was in my late twenties. I walked away from my life in Hollywood, gave everything away, took my clothes off and literally had my 40 days in the desert. I didn't know what I was looking for, but I knew the life I had wasn't fulfilling. What I learned out there, living in pure truth, changed my life forever. I now travel the world showing people how to forever change their lives and never depend on anyone else for their happiness or success. Never get sick again. Start living your purpose. This is true freedom!

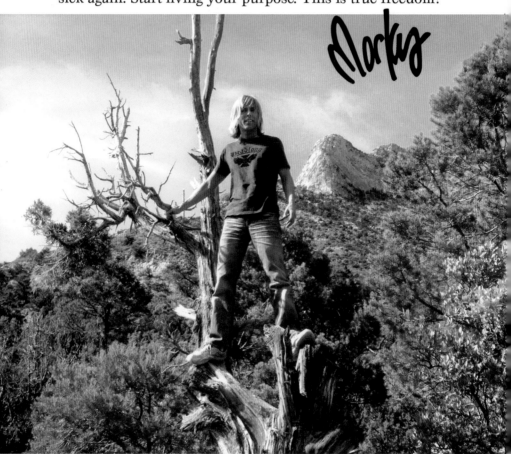

Other Life-changing books, DVDs and products are at:

HealAnything.com

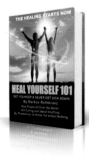
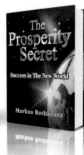
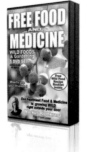
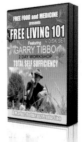
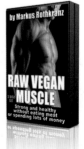
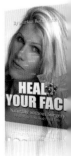